Disinfection for the Home, Home Care, and Ambulatory Care, including Physician Offices

By: Valle C. Oberg

Contents

Introduction

An introduction to the author: My name is Valle C. Oberg. I have worked as a Registered Nurse for the last 22 years now. I began nursing as a Nursing Assistant and home care giver, then received my Practical/Vocational Nursing and on to Registered Nursing. I worked Registry for several years settling down to Intensive Care/Critical Care Transport, then on to Supervision and quite by accident found my true love of Infection Control/Prevention. My then boss Maureen Hanifin coached and guided me to be who I am today. I love Infection Control/Prevention and found my niche so to speak. The past holder of Certification in Infection Control by the CBIC, I love to share my knowledge with others. Sometimes the knowledge is not welcome because new knowledge requires changes in practice and sometimes this is resultant in the increase in Front End Cost. The Back End Cost is always reduced. Always tell your business office or accountant that the Back End Cost (lawsuits, liabilities, increased patient stay, and repeated patient visits) is far more important than the few hundred or even thousand dollars you may need to spend to keep your facility safe.

This book is dedicated to every healthcare professional that wants to use proper cleaning and disinfection techniques. Often, we forget how important the first step of not passing microbes and disease on from person to person. When we are affected, we become angry;

4

however, we all have had lapses in disinfection and cleaning at one point or another. As long as our intent was to do no harm, we can have a clear conscience. If we try to do the right thing, then we are doing the right thing. Any improvement in sanitation practices is a lot better than no improvement.

Basic Microbiology

We cannot truly have good sanitation practices until we know the basics of microbiology. Your organization has the need to maintain a clean, sanitary, healthy environment for the staff, patients, and visitors. The understanding of microbes is the first step of a good infection control program and system. The microbe is an organism that can only be seen with a microscope. Other pathogens or disease producing organisms or their secretions can be seen with the naked eye (depending on your visual acuity).

Microbiology includes the study of, or science of life that is microscopic, or that can be viewed with a microscope. The types of organisms involved are: bacteria, viruses, yeasts, molds, fungi, protozoa, algae, and prions. More detail on these to follow. Microorganisms or those organisms viewable by a microscope are all around us, on our skin, our food, absolutely everywhere. Microorganisms need us and we need them both for survival and to thrive. When a microorganism causes disease, it is called a pathogen or germ.

In order for a microorganism to cause disease in animals or more specifically, humans, it has to gain entrance into our bodies. The ways microorganisms

5

gain entrance are through the nose, eyes, mouth, sweat glands, hair follicles, wounds or other breaks in our skin, by blood or blood products, and through sexual contact. Most commonly it is the nose, mouth, eyes and wounds.

Once entrance to our body is gained, the microorganism grows and multiplies. This growth and multiplication can be very rapid as in cold and flu viruses. It is necessary that it have the right environment for growth and not be killed off by our body's defenses and immune system. Part of this growth is the ability to be transferred to objects and other people by finding an exit route like a sneeze, cough, excrement, and other bodily fluids. Rarely does this happen through sweat glands. The exit route needs other items like water, dust, food, airborne droplets, insects, fomites (inanimate objects), and any other object that the organism can attach itself to for travel to another live object or human.

Bacteria, also called organisms

Bacteria are very small with a few various shapes. Bacteria called cocci are round shaped like berries and can usually be seen under the microscope clumped together. These cocci do good things and bad things. They normally cause infections in the upper respiratory tract including the mouth and throat in the form of streptococcus. On the other hand, staphylococcus causes common infections in the skin, chest, and things like food poisoning.

Bacilli are shaped like a rod being longer than wide and looking like a small rod. Bacilli cause diseases like eye infections, typhoid, diarrhea, pneumonia, salmonella, and even false positive blood infections.

Spirochetes are spiral organisms that kind of look like a corkscrew. Syphilis and trench mouth can be caused by spirochetes. They may be less commonly seen; however, they are truly remarkable under the microscope.

Spores, or spore forming organisms tend to be in the rod shape family. They are stated to be in a resting state until they are activated. The resting state is as it sounds, they are at rest or asleep. When they awaken, the spores produced by the bacteria cause infections and are resistant to normal sanitation, disinfection, and sterilization. These spores are resistant to most cleaning supplies, chemicals, heat, and drying. The spore is very dangerous as it rests or sleeps until the conditions are appropriate for its growth. This makes detection and environmental disinfection a challenge. An example of a spore forming organism is "C-Difficile" or clostridium difficile, a diarrhea producing organism that is involved in significant morbidity (causing disease) and mortality (death). Interestingly enough, the word difficile has the meaning of stubborn or difficult. Difficult to get rid of, that is.

An aerobic organism is an organism that needs oxygen, or what we call air to survive. If the oxygen is removed, the organism dies. Pseudomonas aeruginosa needs oxygen to survive and can live in the soil. This organism needs oxygen and is normally found in areas of the body that are oxygen rich like lungs, blood, and exterior wounds. The yellow-green slime looks nasty and is very difficult to get rid of because it is resistant to most medications. The resistance to antibiotics of pseudomonas in healthcare facilities is presumed to be from the over prescribing of antibiotics and decreased rate of discontinuing the antibiotics that don't work based on cell culture reports. And that is an entirely other issue that is not likely to be solved in the near future.

Anaerobic organisms don't need oxygen to grow, as a matter of fact, they prefer to not have oxygen for growth. We should not buy dented food containing cans because the anaerobic botulism loves to grow without much air. Canned food is harmless because of the way it is canned and heated, killing organisms inside. A dented is a damaged container with the ability of organisms entering the can if there is a puncture in the dent. Once inside, anaerobes can grow and flourish. Tetanus is another anaerobe.

A facultative anaerobe is an anaerobe that has the ability to use oxygen (be aerobic), when oxygen is available. When there is no oxygen, they have the ability to grow as an anaerobe. Salmonella and staphylococcus have this ability.

Organisms reproduce very quickly. An organism is capable of reproducing to over one thousand in number in about two hours under optimum conditions. Luckily, our body's defenses usually can keep them at bay or at least lower their growth rate.

The organism cell wall is permeable or allows through it food that is in a liquefied state. Normally, drying an organism can kill it, or at least diminish its growth capacity. That being said, fomites or inanimate objects do not promote organism growth unless there is a food source in the immediate vicinity of the organism. Like spit on a sidewalk. Usually you don't get sick from it because it dries up relatively quickly and the organism that may be in the spit does not have food, therefore cannot grow or propagate. There are exceptions to every rule.

Gram staining is a method used to assist in the identification of the organism present. An organism that is visible or that absorb the blue dye called crystal violet are called gram positive. If that blue dye can be removed with alcohol and can be stained pink with safranin, they are identified as gram negative organisms. Gram negative organisms are normally found in the intestines.

Just to make the situation a little confusing, there is what is called an acid fast bacilli. These organisms do not succumb to the dye used in gram staining. We need to tell the laboratory to look for AFB or Acid Fast Bacilli so that they can use a special stain called an acid-fast stain. The acid-fast stain turns the cells green. This group of organisms are very difficult to kill. Many disinfectants use this organism group to test their efficacy or effectiveness rating with. Mycobacterium Tuberculosis (TB) in this group.

Organism movement or spread

Organisms move around in a few ways. Organisms can move around by attaching themselves to pieces of dust. Here, they can float around with the hope of entering a susceptible host. The host is like the host of a party.

They allow the organism into the area and introduce them around. Once the organisms find the atmosphere nice, they settle into the party and reproduce.

Organisms can attach themselves to droplets of moisture like a shower head (in the case of legionella and serratia marcescens), or a cough or a sneeze. They travel around on the droplet hoping to find a host so that they can join the party. Serratia is in the pink ring found in toilets and shower heads.

Organisms can be deposited on inanimate objects like door knobs, chairs, clothes, drapes, carpet, tile, counter tops, keyboards, cell phones, pens, pencils, linen, instruments, elevator buttons, shopping carts, and anything else that is not living, a fomite. The organism sits there waiting for a live host to attach to so that they can join the party. After a period of time should there be no host to attach to, the organisms die off. Of special note: organisms are more readily transmitted from a hard non-porous object than from a porous object like drapes and clothes.

Viruses

Viruses are smaller than bacteria with the tendency to be a bit more fragile. Viruses are actually sub-microscopic meaning they require a special microscope (electron microscope) to be seen. Viruses need a host in order to replicate and they die rather rapidly on inanimate objects. They are actually pretty fragile and tend to be easier to kill with the exception of hepatitis.

A Lipophilic virus has a lipid (fat) layer surrounding it. The Lipophilic virus includes the class of Influenza, Human Immunodeficiency Virus (HIV), Respiratory Syncytial Virus (RSV), and a few others.

A Hydrophilic virus don't have the lipid layer and are very difficult to inactivate or kill. Poliovirus, Hepatitis A, and Canine Parvovirus fit this description. The word inactivate is used instead of kill because the virus is inactivated, not killed. By inactivation, it cannot be spread to others.

An Intermediate virus doesn't have a completely lipid coating but has some lipid coating. This means that it is a bit easier than a Hydrophilic virus to inactivate. The Adenovirus and Rotavirus are both in this category.

Fungi

A fungus is much different from viruses and bacteria. More common forms of fungi are mold and mildew. Mushrooms and yeast in bread items are forms of fungus that we eat. The fungi we eat is not harmful. Fungi cause disease in skin, lungs, and mucus membranes mostly. The athlete's foot fungus Trichophyton is used by companies in testing disinfectants. As you know from attempting to get rid of bathroom mildew, it can be tough to get rid of.

Protozoa

Although not necessarily a large concern to healthcare facilities. Protozoa is mentioned here so that we can learn how to prevent their spread. Protozoa is single celled and living.

Waterborne diseases like giardia involve protozoa. Giardia is spread through fecal – oral contact. Cleaning and hygiene are very important to stop the spread of certain protozoa.

Prions

Probably the toughest of the tough is the prion. Prions affect the brain causing the deterioration of brain tissue. The most widely known prion is responsible for the Mad Cow Disease and scrapie in sheep. Prions are composed of protein, making the transformation into an abnormal protein that accumulates and causes disease.

Prions and instruments that have been infected with prions need special processing as prions are resistant to normal sterilization. There are some recommendations for a 1:2 dilution of bleach or N sodium hydroxide for a time period of over one hour. Most instruments will be greatly damaged with this high of a concentration of bleach as they will corrode.

Vectors and others

Let's not forget the vectors and other methods of travel of certain microorganisms. Animals, birds, mosquitoes, and other insects can help travel of microorganisms and even have a few of their own. Psittacosis is often associated with bird droppings from pigeons. West Nile Virus and malaria from mosquitoes and Lyme disease from tics, just to name a few.

General control of microorganisms

Light

Sunlight is wonderful and natural for disinfecting items. Light from the sun is not dependable and cannot be depended on for disinfection. Some health facilities are using ultraviolet light to rid the air of bacteria and other microorganisms. The downside of ultraviolet light is that it cannot penetrate objects. It is under experimentation though to see what it can accomplish.

Cold

Cold, meaning temperature cold and not the cold that is catchy, inhibits or slows the growth of organisms. We use cold when we refrigerate and freeze food. Frozen food will still have degradation, but not to the degree as food left out. The organism is inhibited from growth by the cold allowing us to save food for long periods of time prior to cooking.

Heat

Heat can inactivate and kill all microorganisms. A higher than usual heat can even inactivate prions. Spore forming organisms are used to determine the effectiveness of disinfection and sterilization. Heat is used both as moist and dry in the pasteurization, disinfection, and sterilization process.

Chemicals

Chemicals of different types are used in the inactivation and destruction of microorganisms. Some chemicals disinfect, while others sanitize. We use chemicals every day to clean our homes and work spaces. Choosing the right chemical requires a bit of education so as to render the microorganisms harmless while protecting the integrity of the item being cleaned.

Sanitization kills only disease producing organisms where disinfection kills most organisms.

An antiseptic is a chemical that prevents growth of microorganisms on the human body. Some soaps contain antiseptics and some creams and other cosmetic items contain antiseptics. Hand sanitizer is an antiseptic.

Disinfectants are also called germicidal or bactericidal, even though there is a bit of a difference between the three. Disinfectants work on microorganisms on a surface that is not living. Disinfectants are often too harsh or even toxic to the human body, thus making them dangerous if not used properly.

Bacteriostatic agents inhibit the growth of organism without necessarily killing them. Bacteriostats essentially keep microorganisms from multiplying. Bacteriostats are used in some antibiotics, cleaning products for the home and in cosmetics.

Sanitizing refers to the killing of bacteria and some viruses to render them harmless. It reduces the numbers of the microorganisms so that the number is so few that it will not create illness.

Sterilizing is the complete destruction of all microorganisms including spores, bacteria, viruses, and fungi. Sterilizing here does not refer to prions, they are a special case.

Preservatives inhibit microbial growth in food, drugs, cosmetics and other household products.

Cobalt Radiation can sterilize items also. It is not used in a widespread manner in the United States by hospitals, it is used to sterilize disposable medical equipment.

Gas is used to sterilize in hospitals also. Mostly the very large hospitals and even some dental offices use EtO or Ethylene Oxide gas to sterilize instruments.

Bacterial Counts

Bacterial counts are used to identify the severity of infections and how well a disinfectant or cleaning agent work. When evaluating the effectiveness of a disinfectant or sanitizer, organism counts are important. Organism counts are taken over several areas of the surface being studied before and after the disinfection or cleaning method is used. This way we can find the effectiveness of a product or method of cleaning. Organism counts are used by laboratories with fluid or tissue cultures to tell the physician how many organisms are present. This way, the physician can order the appropriate treatment and even evaluate if it is a true infection, or are they just present just hanging around. Organism counts are not used on viruses. Polymerase Chain Reaction (PCR) testing is used instead to identify that the virus is present by looking at the

Deoxyribonucleic Acid (DNA) and Ribonucleic Acid (RNA). Sometimes PCR testing can give a colony count of the organisms.

Bacteria hang around in clumps. When cleaning, the clumps may be broken up and the organism are redistributed in an area, thus beginning to grow in new clumps. This may produce higher organism counts when talking about cleaning methods and supplies. The cleaning supplies are easily contaminated making it possible to inadvertently spread microorganisms from one place to the next.

Governmental Involvement

The government regulates agents involved in microbial activity destruction or inhibition. Medical facilities need to use methods that are approved by the appropriate governmental agency.

The Environmental Protection Agency (EPA) is responsible for protecting human health and the safeguarding of the environment such as air, water, and land. The EPA operates under the Federal Insecticide, Fungicide and Rodenticide Act (FIFRA). The FIFRA outlines regulations in the use of pesticides, registration of pesticides, manufacture of pesticides, and pesticide safety and effectiveness. FIFRA defines a pesticide as any substance intended in preventing, destroying, repelling, or mitigating any pest, and any substance or mix of substances intended for use as insecticides, herbicides, fungicides, rodenticides, disinfectants, sanitizers, plant regulators, defoliants or desiccants. That being said, there is EPA registration for disinfectants, sanitizers, and other items because they destroy microorganisms or inhibit their growth. The EPA website has the data on all of these items under pesticide.

Claims on labels of pesticides need to meet certain criteria.

Limited/Minimal Disinfection Claim for germicides, disinfectants, and bactericides means they are recommended for limited use against gram positive or gram negative bacteria only. The label must state it is against gram positive or gram negative bacteria and is tested on salmonella and staphylococcus.

Hospital General Use Disinfectants for medical and dental use are tested with staphylococcus, salmonella and pseudomonas aeruginosa.

Food Preparation Area Sanitizers are tested with escherichia coli and staphylococcus.

Sanitizers for non-food contact surfaces are tested against staphylococcus and klebsiella pneumonia or enterobacter aerogenes.

A Tuberculocidal claim means that the product kills Mycobacteria Tuberculosis, it may be tested on the variant Mycobacteria Bovis (cows). Humans can acquire TB from cattle and other animals, although it is rare.

Fungicidal claim means the chemical kills Trichophyton mentagrophytes, or Athlete's Foot.

How to read the EPA registration number:

The first three numbers are the EPA manufacturer assigned number.

The next number(s) is the EPA registered product number.

The last number(s) is the EPA company number of the distributor of the product.

United States Department of Agriculture (USDA)

The USDA has a hand in chemicals also. Chemicals that are used around food processing plants that include cleaning agents, sanitizers, and lubricants that can have incidental contact with food are regulated by the USDA.

USDA category codes:

A1 – Compounds used for general cleaning on all surfaces.

Prior to using the compound, all food and packaging must be protected or removed from the area. After use, surfaces must be thoroughly rinsed with potable (drinkable) water.

A2 – Compounds for use only in soak tanks or with steam or mechanical cleaning devices.

A3 – Acid cleaners.

Prior to using the compound, all food and packaging must be protected or removed from the area. After use, surfaces must be thoroughly rinsed with potable water.

A4 – Floor and wall cleaners.
Prior to using the compound, all food and packaging must be protected or removed from the area. After use, surfaces must be thoroughly rinsed with potable water.

A6 – Scouring cleaners.
All odors or abrasive residue must be removed prior to using the cleaned surface for direct food contact.

A7 – Metal cleaners and polishes meant for non-food contact surfaces.

A8 – Degreasers or carbon removers for food cooking or smoking equipment, utensils,   or other surfaces associated with food cooking or smoking. Prior to using the
compound, all food and packaging must be protected or removed from the area.
After use, surfaces must be thoroughly rinsed with potable water. All odors must be removed prior to reprocessing food products.

C1 – Compounds for use on surfaces in inedible non-processing area.
Products in this category are odor controlling products, sanitizers, paint removers, cleaning and sanitizing

products with strong odors or perfume including pine oil. If these products are used on items to be returned to food processing areas. All surfaces must be thoroughly rinsed with potable water.

C1 – General products. They are evaluated on a case-by-case basis only.

C2 – Toilet and dressing room supplies.

D1 – Antimicrobial agents that require rinsing. Disinfectants used on hard nonporous surfaces, including utensils must be followed by a potable water rinse.

D2 – Antimicrobial agents not requiring rinsing. Sanitizing solutions that are formulated in compliance with other regulations may be used on surfaces without regard to rinsing.

E1 – Hand washing products that do not contain perfumes or leave a residual odor on hands after rinsing.

E4 – Hand creams, powders, and lotions can be used by employees at the end of the day in areas that are not meant for processing of food.

L1 – General drain and sewer cleaners.

P1 – Other products.

Q1 – Egg shell cleaning products require a warm potable water rinse after use.

Q3 – Egg shell sanitizers must be quaternary ammonium products for use after cleaning
    and rinsed with potable water thoroughly if the egg shell is damaged in any way;
    otherwise, no rinsing necessary.

The EPA has what are called signal words for the potency of products. The Lethal Dose (LD) of the product guides the use of the word on the label.

- Danger-Poison
    - LD is less than 50mg/kg ingested substance, or
    - Product is corrosive or produces irreversible damage to skin, or
    - Product is corrosive to ocular tissue or corneal irritation beyond 21 days
- Warning
    - LD is between 50-500mg/kg ingested substance, or
    - Product causes severe redness or swelling at three days, or
    - Product corneal involvement or irritation clears 8-21 days
- Caution

- o Harmful is between 500-5000mg/kg ingested, or
  - o Product causes moderate redness at three days, or
  - o Product corneal involvement clears within 7 days
- Caution (optional)
  - o 5000mg/kg is not harmful if ingested, or
  - o Product causes slight or no irritation at three days, or
  - o Product causes minimal irritation to eye that clears within 24 hours

Food and Drug Administration (FDA)

The FDA is responsible for the safety of our food supply and the safety of the chemicals that come in contact with our food supply and in retail food establishments. The FDA publishes the standards and requirements for the proper cleaning and sanitizing of surfaces that come in contact with food. However, State and Local governments are responsible for the inspections of these food establishments.

The FDA has the additional fiduciary responsibility to regulate medical devices and their accessories. Liquid chemical germicides are seen from the FDA's viewpoint as an accessory also. Liquid chemical germicides include sterilants and disinfectants.

The FDA also regulates over the counter items like hand sanitizers and antimicrobial soaps. Surgical scrub and surgical skin antiseptics are also included in this group.

Occupational Safety and Health Administration (OSHA)

OSHA is primarily concerned with the health and welfare of the work force. Recently, OSHA is overlapping into the infection control practices of healthcare facilities.

The CFR (Code of Federal Regulations), we usually hear about in the healthcare setting is 1910.1030 or the blood borne pathogen regulation. It was meant to protect the worker from exposure to blood and other potentially infectious materials. Other potentially infectious materials includes bodily fluids and tissues. OSHA has expanded this very recently to include sterilization and infection control standards in order to minimize the exposure to the worker during the practice of disinfection and sterilization.

Not being absolutely sure of the reason for this recent change, it can be presumed to be because many of the dental and outpatient clinics are not regulated by any other sources except the business license. An example of this was the endoscopy clinic crisis in Las Vegas, Nevada. The only way the one clinic was shut down for poor infection control practices was that the mayor Oscar Goodman removed their business license; therefore, they could not be open as a business while the investigation continued.

OSHA also has several other standards that apply to businesses including the workplace and worker right to know what hazards are present in the workplace, CFR 1910.1200.

Centers for Disease Control and Prevention (CDC)

The CDC is the lead or top agency that's purpose is to protect the health and welfare of people here in the United States, and worldwide. The CDC develops and applies the prevention and control of diseases and has activities that promotes and educates with the purpose to improve the health of people in the United States. The CDC develops guidelines for the use of germicides and other infection prevention activities.

Disinfectants and Sanitizing Agents

Cleaning will be discussed a bit later; however, a very important point is to be made here. No matter what the surface, it cannot be sanitized, disinfected, or sterilized when it has not been cleaned first. Chemicals, heat, and gas for use in sanitization, disinfection, and sterilization cannot penetrate dirt or other organic or non-organic debris or biofilm. Biofilm is a matrix substance made up of protein, fat, and organisms that form on an item or instrument. Chemicals and other means of disinfection, sanitization, and sterilization cannot penetrate this layer or biofilm. This is why it is so important to soak instruments soon after use and clean thoroughly before any attempt at disinfection or sterilization.

One note: bleach is probably one of the very few substances that can eat through biofilm once it is there. Bleach is very corrosive to instruments and supplies making it not desirable to use for this purpose. Use bleach to get biofilm out of animal water dishes and rinse the dishes thoroughly prior to allowing the animal to drink out of it. That method of biofilm removal with bleach is completely acceptable. An alternative is to clean animal dishes with vinegar.

The dwell time of a chemical agent is the amount of time the chemical needs to sit on the surface before the organism/viruses are inactivated/killed. The dwell time is important because the disinfectant needs to remain on the surface for that amount of time prior to rinsing or using the equipment again. It makes a huge difference in room and equipment turnover time. Always refer to manufacturer data when making the decision as to the dwell time of a product. Most often though, it is ten minutes.

Phenolics

Phenolics have been around for the disinfection of surfaces in hospitals and clinics for a very long time. Phenolics carry a tuberculocidal claim which makes them widely used in medical care facilities. Phenolics have been mixed with detergents to make them good cleaner-disinfectants. They cannot be used with non-ionic synthetic detergents because the detergents will render the phenolics useless. If a cleaner-disinfectant is desired, purchase a chemical that is created for that purpose. Phenolics are more alkaline so mixing would only be in accordance with manufacturer's instructions.

Phenolics have been associated with increasing the bilirubin levels in newborns. This is especially important when cleaning bassinettes as they can cause hyperbilirubinemia in infants.. The recommendation is to use something other than a phenolic. There is no worry if the phenolic is rinsed off the bassinette after the required dwell time.

Quaternary Ammoniums (Quats)

This class of disinfectant only recently became available over the counter at a bit of a lesser concentration than medical facilities can use. Different formulations of quats are used for different germicidal activities. They are very good and can be used in nurseries without the concern of hyperbilirubinemia in newborns. Quats can be used in food establishments also. Quats are more alkaline so mixing would only be in accordance with manufacturer's instructions.

Acid Disinfectants

Acid disinfectants also clean by changing the chemistry of the environment. Acids make it very difficult for microbes to reproduce and live. Vinegar is one good acid; however, it does not have stable properties for disinfection so cannot be used in facilities. Sometimes the quats are added to the acids to improve the germicidal actions.

Iodine

Iodophors which are iodines combined with non-ionic synthetic detergents are touted as iodine products, but they actually have less negative characteristics than straight iodine. Iodine scrubs for surgical applications fit this description. Acids are combined with idophors in order to make them more germicidal. Phosphoric acid or hydrochloric acid are usually used. With the additional acidity, iodophors or iodine solutions can be a bit corrosive. When iodine containing preparations are used on patient's skin, a careful look into seafood or iodine allergy would be prudent as the reactions can be quite severe. Iodophors can permanently stain some materials with blue or rust stains. The blue staining is on starched fabrics.

Chlorine

Chlorine is a wonderful disinfectant, with properties that make it undesirable for certain surfaces and textiles. When all else fails, we turn to chlorine. The well-known solution of freshly prepared (that day), one part chlorine to ten parts water is the standard disinfection in most areas. That being said, chlorine or sodium hypochlorite is unstable in the presence of light, heat, or organic soil. As those with pools know, adding chlorine is a common task because it evaporates rather easily and is dissipated by light. That is why what we call, "shocking" (adding more chlorine immediately prior to swimming in a pool or spa) is necessary. And the stronger smell of the chlorine does not indicate powerfulness because the body oils, soil, and dirt make much of the available chlorine ineffective. Today's pools use more bromine than chlorine. The bromine and other chemicals that are not natural make the water non-potable.

Chlorine is corrosive and damaging to steel, carpet fiber, clothing and skin. If chlorine is accidentally spilled on your skin, a slimy feel results. That slimy feel is the chlorine damaging your skin and needs to be rinsed off immediately. Chlorine is alkaline and should never ever be mixed with any other chemicals, especially acidic chemicals. The gas cloud is noxious and damaging to airways.

Gluteraldehyde (Glut pronounced Gloot)

Gluteraldehyde is quickly becoming less widely used because of the carcinogen effects it has been found to have. Gluteraldehyde is a cold sterilant for instruments that are sensitive to heat.
Gluteraldehyde is to be used on general surfaces for cleaning and disinfecting. Gluteraldehydes require special handling and room ventilation.

Glycols

Glycols are used in air sanitization products. A solution of 5-10% glycol is required to be considered an air sanitizer. Some facilities are using this to disinfect entire rooms.

Silver

Ionic silver has been used for years in burn creams. Some burn creams have a combination of silver and sulfur compounds. Even though silver's efficacy is variable, it is proving to be a weapon against infections in healthcare facilities. Silver is now being used in many healthcare items ranging from Foley catheters, intravenous catheters, and wound dressings. Many people confuse silver allergy and nickel allergy. Most jewelry allergy is actually to nickel as true silver allergy is rare. Beware though that you should be aware of the silver contained products in your facility because although rare, an ionic silver allergy can be deadly.

Antimicrobial hand soap

These products in health care facilities often have PCMX (chloroxylenol) or Triclosan in them. PCMX is a good hand sanitizer; however, not labeled for use otherwise. PCMX tends to cause more skin irritation than Triclosan or just plain soap and water. Companies that have hand soaps with PCMX often combine the PCMX with lotions and emollients in an attempt to decrease the skin irritation.

Triclosan is a widely used hand antimicrobial and can be found both in over the counter toothpaste, acne creams, hand preparations and in healthcare facilities. Recent data shows that triclosan has been found in the water supply and in users' bloodstream indicating absorption through the skin. Some organism resistance has also been associated with triclosan.

For hand antisepsis, plain soap and water are just fine EXCEPT in surgical suites and other areas where germ-free environments are necessary.

Nitti Gritty Guide

With the background and basics covered, we will now enter the material that most people are looking for. The easiest to understand guide to disinfection and sterilization for all healthcare types from the Acute Care Hospital to Assisted Living and even your own home.

As an Infection Control/Prevention Practitioner, the need to be in a sanitary environment cannot be overstressed. If our homes are a sloppy and dirty mess, so tends to be our habits at work. Sometimes, a look at someone's car including in the windows can give an indication on our priorities regarding our physical environment, or how busy they are. People with cluttered cars often have cluttered homes. People with cars that have open food wrappers and other items strewn about tend not to have the best hygienic practices that tend to spill over into the work environment. There are always exceptions to everything as there are a few people that have wonderful work practices and their homes and cars are a mess.

Preventing infection from sources of medical invasive tests and procedures is of the utmost importance. It is in the news on an almost weekly basis that some clinic or hospital has to test hundreds of patients because they had lapses in infection control standards. These lapses range from inadequate disinfection and sterilization techniques to re-using syringes and needles. We, in the medical field know better. Sometimes we get used to sloppy practices and sometimes it is to save money. I urge everyone that reads this book to use the information wisely and do onto others as you would like done onto you.

The documented infections from inadequately disinfected and sterilized equipment range from tuberculosis and hepatitis to pseudomonas. Most often, lapses in infection control standards lead to the transmission of the more hearty organisms as the weak ones tend to die off quickly.

Cleaning

Cleaning is the physical removal of dirt and debris from objects. The process of cleaning also removes pathogens, or disease producing microorganisms. Cleaning does not remove everything making further processing necessary for certain items.

The physical action of cleaning can involve manual or mechanical methods and supplies ranging from brushes to machines. Items must be cleaned before they can be disinfected or sterilized. This cannot be emphasized enough. Chemicals cannot do their work with biofilm and other organic or inorganic matter in the way.

Decontamination

Decontamination is the process of removing pathogenic or disease causing microorganisms from objects or surfaces so that they are safe to handle, use, or discard. In the instance of sterilization or disinfection, many times items are decontaminated during the cleaning process and sometimes before.

Cidal

The term cidal or cide means it has killing action associated with the chemical in use. Cidal is used at the end of the word and generally indicates that the chemical will kill pathogenic microorganisms.

Disinfection

Disinfection eliminates most of or all pathogenic microorganisms (except bacterial spores) on inanimate objects. Different levels of disinfection are necessary depending on the type of use an item or instrument is meant for. Liquid chemicals are the most common type of liquid disinfection in healthcare facilities in the United States.

Levels of disinfection

High level disinfection will kill all microorganisms except large amounts of bacterial spores.

Intermediate level disinfection may kill mycoorganisms like TB, vegetative (receives nutrients from soil) organisms, most viruses, most fungi, but not bacterial spores.

Low level disinfection can kill most vegetative bacteria, some viruses, and some fungi, usually in ten minutes or less.

Sterilization

Sterilization is the method used to rid objects of all viable microorganisms and bacterial spores. Bacterial spores are used as one of the methods used to evaluate the effectiveness of sterilization.

Spaulding Method description

Earle Spaulding devised an approach to disinfection and sterilization of patient-care items and equipment. This method is so clear and makes so much sense that it has been adopted into general use throughout the medical community. It actually makes very good sense because the level of disinfection or sterilization is based on the degree of risk of infection that could occur with the use of an instrument or equipment. Three classifications are used, Critical, Semicritical, and Noncritical.

Critical Items

Critical items in the Spaulding classification system refer to a high risk of infection should they become contaminated with any microorganism. These items enter normally sterile body tissue. This makes it critical that the items be sterile.

Critical items include surgical instruments, vascular catheters, cardiac catheters, urinary catheters, implants, and anything else that enters normally sterile tissue or compartments.

> Laparoscopes and arthroscopes that enter normally sterile tissue should be sterilized between patients. This does not always occur, and at times high level disinfection is used because of the difficulty in cleaning the intricate parts of the device. Newer items can be safely sterilized (refer to manufacturer's instructions). Even though they are critical items, no infections have been reported from the proper use of high level disinfection of these instruments instead of sterilization.

Critical items need absolute sterilization by the method that is recommended by the device manufacturer. Never reuse an item that was meant to be a single use item. Sterilizing single use items can cause breakdown of the materials the item was made with making it easier for microorganisms to get into the areas making structural injury of the object.

Semicritical Items

Semicritical items come in contact with mucous membranes or nonintact skin. The chances for infection from microorganism transmission are high, but not as high as for critical items. Mucous membranes are generally resistant to infection by bacterial spores, mycoorganisms, and viruses.

Examples of Semicritical items are laryngoscope blades, cystoscopes, diaphragm fitting rings, respiratory therapy equipment, some endoscopes, and anesthesia equipment.

Noncritical items

Noncritical items come in contact with intact skin or potentially nonintact skin, but come in contact with nonintact skin only for a short time. Noncritical items include bed side rails, hydrotherapy tanks, blood pressure cuffs, stethoscopes, some electronic thermometers, wheelchairs, chairs, computers, pens, pencils, and many others.

The CDC says there is virtually no risk of spread of infection through these devices; however, private journals implicate them in transmission.

As a note: hydrotherapy tanks and foot soaks at beauty salons have been implicated in transmission of infection. Some facilities have changed the cleaning of these items to bleach because of the fungus that can be transmitted.

The disinfectants approved for noncritical items have a dwell time of about ten minutes. Even with this documentation, the CDC states that multiple investigators have demonstrated that these disinfectants are effective against many bacteria, viruses, and candida with exposure times of only 30-60 seconds. That being said, always refer to manufacturer's instructions in the proper use of any product.

Disinfection for the Home, Home Care, and Ambulatory Care, including Physician Offices

The need to disinfect in all areas of care is necessary to curtail the spread of infections. Patients in the home are now as ill as they used to be in the hospitals. Thirty years ago and prior, patients could spend a few days in the hospital for a very thorough physical exam. Patients would remain in the hospital waiting for tests and routine procedures. This is no more, patients are sent home sooner and remain at home for procedures and tests that are now performed in outpatient areas. These patients may have invasive devices, immunocompromising conditions, and even communicable diseases.

The patient recovering at home should have a less risk at acquiring an infection than in the hospital or healthcare setting. This is because hospitals and other healthcare settings allow for the transmission of pathogens through inadequate sanitation, disinfection, and sterilization. Epidemics are easily curtailed if people stay in their homes. Specific examples of disinfection needs follow.

Reusable devices such as crutches, blood pressure cuffs, and other items that only touch intact skin can be cleaned only with a detergent. EPA registered low-level and intermediate-level disinfectants are perfect for this purpose. The detergents that are appropriate are EPA registered and some are available over the counter. Three percent hydrogen peroxide has been shown to disinfect room drapes when sprayed on stains or areas where organisms are present.

Even though germs don't jump, they are deposited on the floors of healthcare institutions and can then travel via wheelchairs, gurneys, beds, shoes, and other objects.

> Caution against the use of the following solutions for healthcare needs or disinfection in the home:
> - Vinegar
> - Baking soda
> - Borax
> - Ammonia

Reusable devices such as Tracheostomy tubes –
1. 70% isopropyl alcohol soak for 5 minutes, or
2. Hydrogen peroxide 3% soak for 30 minutes, or
3. 1:50 dilution of 5.25-6.15% sodium hypochlorite (bleach) soak for 5 minutes

Mops

Mops and cloths used to clean healthcare facilities need cleaned and disinfected on a routine basis. Routine laundering is acceptable on a daily basis. The water used for the mops and cloths also needs to be changed every three to four rooms and at least every 60 minutes. Mopping can increase the spread of microbes throughout the facility. The cleaning cloths that are not clean also spreads microbes rather rapidly. Spot cleaning with a disposable towel that is impregnated with a disinfectant is okay for non-critical surfaces. Many facilities are switching to disposable antimicrobial mop heads and other products.

Endoscopes

Endoscopes are difficult to clean. They have long channels that can trap water, viruses, and organisms. Although the risk of acquiring an infection from an endoscope is rare, it does happen.

Part of the cleaning process with endoscopes is flushing after cleaning. The flushing can be done with sterile water, filtered water, or tap water. The rinsing rids the scope of debris and residue left over from the disinfection process. The residue from the disinfectants has resulted in disinfectant induced colitis in the past. Scopes rinsed with sterile water decrease risk of transmission of organisms that can be found in tap water like pseudomonas, legionella and mycobacteria. A non-sterile water rinse should be followed by an alcohol rinse and forced air drying. Forced air drying is necessary to reduce organism contamination when the scopes are stored.

When the processing and drying of endoscopes is completed, they should be dried and stored in a way that prevents recontamination. Hanging the scopes works well as long as they don't touch each other or any part of the cabinet they are in.

Scopes

Heat stable scopes should be steam sterilized. When unable to be steam sterilized, cold sterilization with chemicals is appropriate and may be faster. Scopes that are used in endoscopic procedures or other semi-critical (contact with mucus membranes) that are also used with other equipment such as biopsy forceps or other items for use in normally sterile areas can be high-level disinfected as long as the tool used with the scope is sterile. This is remembering that high-level disinfected scopes when properly cleaned, disinfected, and dried are rid of all microorganisms except spores. To date, no infections from spores have been documented.

All heat sensitive scopes must be properly cleaned, followed by a minimum of high-level disinfection. A few products for this purpose have been stated to cause damage to scopes because of the oxidation and coloring of lens. Proper cleaning often prevents the discoloration of scope lenses from disinfection chemicals. Use only those disinfectants that have been FDA approved for the scope and always abide by manufacturer recommendations.

The very first step of disinfection of any object, scopes included is cleaning. Scopes are more difficult to clean because of the long lumens and size of the lumens. Clean meticulously, regardless of the time that may be involved. Cleaning begins at the bedside. Some automatic endoscope reprocessors are now FDA approved to include the cleaning process. Even so, nothing takes away from the initial cleaning that begins at the bedside that is necessary.

Development of protective barriers and sheaths is ongoing. The barriers that are in use now may decrease the associated risk for infection from improperly cleaned or disinfected scopes. The new capsule camera that can be swallowed is not a replacement for endoscopy as biopsy's cannot be performed from the camera. They do give a look at what is going on, but cannot replace the diagnostic efficacy of an endoscopy.

Training is essential for endoscopy personnel. Too many times training has been you show me and I will show others. This type of training leads to miscommunication, misunderstanding, and misutilization of equipment. The training should be from an accredited agency and performed initially and on at minimum, a yearly basis.

Steps of endoscope disinfection/sterilization with liquid chemicals all have a few basic steps.

1. At the bedside and after the procedure is complete, endoscopes are generally wiped off

2. After the endoscope is wiped off, the channels are rinsed with an enzymatic detergent
3. The endoscope is transported to the processing department in a manner that prevents injury or contamination of other items or areas
4. Mechanically clean the external surfaces and internal surfaces which includes brushing internal channels and flushing the internal channels with water and an enzymatic cleaner or detergent
5. Leak test the scope prior to immersion
6. Disinfect the scope using the appropriate high-level disinfectant
   a. Always follow manufacturer's instructions
   b. Immerse the endoscope in the high-level disinfectant or use a chemical sterilant and instill the chemicals in all of the channels to avoid air pockets
   c. Soak the scope for the recommended time period
7. Rinse the endoscope and purge all of the channels with preferably sterile water, or can use filtered water or tap water that meets federal water standards for clean water
8. Purge all channels with alcohol
9. Purge all channels with dry forced air (follow manufacturer guidelines as to Pressure Per Square Inch (PSI) that can be used with each particular scope
10. Store endoscopes in a manner that promotes drying and prevents contamination
    a. Hung vertically in a ventilated cabinet
       i. If scopes leak onto floor, they were not dry prior to hanging

1. Many surveyors are now being taught to look at the bottom of the cabinets for evidence of wet scopes
ii. Scopes should not touch each other
iii. Scopes should not touch the cabinet
b. Scopes can be stored in ventilated cases that are disinfected
11. Transport scopes within and outside facility in impermeable disinfected cases
a. Cases used for transportation outside the facility should not be used inside
i. If a dirty scope is put in the case, the case should be destroyed
12. Keep scopes that are clean in a separate room from those that are dirty
13. Final rinse water used if not sterile should be cultured on a monthly basis
a. Monthly water cultures for the facility should be sufficient

Laparoscopes, arthroscopes and any other scope that enters normally sterile tissue should be sterilized for optimum results; however, high-level disinfection may suffice according to the CDC when sterilization is not feasible.

Vaginal probes and endocavitary probes contact mucus membranes only. They should have a condom or probe cover for each use and changed between patients. Even though probe covers may be in use, the probes need high-level disinfection. Many of the companies that make the probes also make or recommend specific disinfection systems. As a tidbit of information, probe covers have a very high perforation rate, whereas condoms do not.

If your manufacturer recommends 2% gluteraldehyde, see if they can recommend an alternate method of high-level disinfection because gluteraldehyde can shorten the life of the transducer and also can be detrimental on human gametes and embryos if not rinsed off to remove all residual chemical.

The CDC offers an alternative procedure:
1. Mechanical removal of gel from transducer
2. Cleaning the transducer in soap and water
3. Wiping the transducer in 70% alcohol
   a. Alternatively soak 1-2 minutes in 500 ppm chlorine
4. Rinsing with tap water
5. Air dry

Ultrasound probes used during surgical procedures need to have a sterile sheath used over the probe. The probe itself needs to be sterilized between cases. If the entire probe is not immersible, the tip of the probe can be high-level disinfected with the rest by immersion in the chemicals or wrapping in a cloth saturated with the high-level disinfectant for the appropriate amount of time. Always rinse with tap water and dry after disinfection.

Dental Instrumentation

Sterilization is necessary for instruments and items that normally penetrate soft tissue or bone
1. Scalpel blades
2. Bone chisels
3. Periodontal scalers
4. Extraction forceps
5. Surgical burs
6. Any other instrument that penetrates soft tissue or bone

Sterilization is recommended; however, high-level disinfection is acceptable for heat sensitive instruments that come in contact with oral tissues
1. Air syringes
2. Water syringes
3. Amalgam condensers
4. And others

Hand pieces should be heat sterilized after each patient. If they cannot be heat sterilized, get rid of them and purchase some that can.

High touch surfaces are those that are frequently touched with gloved and ungloved hands during patient care. It is separated from non-contact or housekeeping surfaces because the clinical surfaces have the possibility of becoming contaminated when gloved hands have blood or other potentially infectious material on them.

High touch surfaces include these items in clinical areas:

1. Light switches
2. Chair switches
3. X-ray equipment
4. Chair side computers
5. Any other area in the immediate clinical area

Clinical areas can have barrier precautions used when feasible such as a clear plastic covering over the surface or item. The plastic barrier should be changed between patients, when soiled or damaged. If no barrier is used, the items should be disinfected with an intermediate disinfectant with a tuberculocidal claim or low-level disinfected with a disinfectant that has a claim for hospital use or HBV (Hepatitis B Virus) and HIV (Human Immunodeficiency Virus) claim.

The housekeeping surfaces can be cleaned with detergent and water or a hospital disinfectant. If contaminated, the surface should be cleaned with a hospital disinfectant after being cleaned properly.

Hemodialysis

Hemodialysis is one of the most common methods of acquiring bloodborne viruses and organisms from others. Both the FDA and EPA regulate the disinfectants for reprocessing the hemodialyzers and hemodialysis machines and their water treatment systems.

Due to the large amount of bloodborne pathogens that can be transmitted at a dialysis center because of the nature of the treatment, the non-critical surfaces need to be disinfected with EPA registered disinfectants. The non-critical surfaces are items such as chairs, counters, scissors, hemostats, clamps, blood pressure cuffs, stethoscopes, and the outside of the dialysis machines. If any non-critical item is contaminated with visible blood, then a disinfectant with a tuberculocidal, HBV, or HIV claim should be used to decontaminate the item. Alternatively, a solution of 1:100 parts bleach (sodium hypochlorite) to water can be used.

The guidelines for the dialysis centers help maintain a clean and sanitary environment so that the chances of transmission of pathogens are negligible.

The mode of disinfection in dialysis centers is usually with paracetic acid, glutaraldehyde, heat pasteurization, or a chlorine method. The entire system for dialysis is usually cleaned with a chlorine containing compound or heat pasteurization. It is an exception, however to also use formaldehyde paracetic acid or ozone. In our area heat disinfection is often used for dialysis machines. Most often paracetic acid is often used to re-process the dialyzer. Although glutaraldehyde is still used it's not very common due to the fumes and exposure risks.

Hepatitis B surface antigen positive patients should have their dialysis at the end of the day. The machine needs to be heat treated before the next patient, alternatively the machine can be chemically treated.

Sterilization

Critical items have to be sterilized between uses. Machine and chemical sterilization methods can be used. Heat and moisture sensitive items can be sterilized with chemicals like hydrogen peroxide gas plasma, peracetic acid, and ethylene oxide. Most hospitals don't use ethylene oxide, the larger medical centers may.

Steam sterilization uses moist heat of saturated steam under pressure. This is the most widely used method of sterilization in hospitals and doctor offices. The machines come in all sizes and are basically dependable and easy to take care of. This method of sterilization is pretty inexpensive for its purpose. Steam sterilization is accomplished with steam, pressure, temperature, and time. The pressure is used to get to the high temperature that is necessary to quickly kill microorganisms.

One type of steam sterilization is the gravity displacement autoclave that puts in steam at the top or the sides of the chamber and with steam being lighter than air, it forces air out of the bottom of the camber through a vent.

The other type of sterilization is pre-vacuum which has a vacuum pump that makes sure the air is removed from the chamber before the steam is allowed in.

Both use a test called Bowie-Dick that can detect air leaks. An air leak would make the entire load of items to be sterilized unsterile. The Bowie-Dick is placed in the center of a pack and run in an empty load. This test is done at the beginning of the day before any sterilization takes place.

Sterilizers should be tested with mechanical, biological and chemical means. This cannot be stressed enough.

Flash Sterilization

"Flash" steam sterilization is sterilization of an unwrapped object at 132 degrees Celsius for 3 minutes at 27-28 lbs. of pressure in a gravity displacement sterilizer. The time required for flash sterilization depends on the type of sterilizer and the type of item. Flash sterilization should only be used as an emergent means of sterilizing an instrument that has been dropped in the middle of a procedure. It should not be used as a routine method of sterilization. Refer to your sterilizers instructions on how to perform flash sterilization. Remember to clean the item first. Also be careful not to burn yourself or the patient when using instruments that were, "flashed". There are special packages made just for flashing items, the trays are made just for that purpose, just don't overload the tray. When the unavoidable flashing of an implant occurs, keep a log of the item, date, time, biological indicator results, and the patient it was used on.

Low-Temperature Sterilization

Ethylene oxide (ETO) is used as one of the low-temperature sterilants. It will usually be seen in larger medical centers. Some supplies are very sensitive to heat, so they need to be sterilized with low temperatures and ETO supplies that need. Other gases are also used also.

Peracetic acid is used as a cold immersion technique along with gluteraldehyde. Hydrogen peroxide is also being used as a gas, ionizing radiation, ultraviolet light and chlorine dioxide are in use also.

Preparation for sterilization

Most facilities wrap their items in trays that are double wrapped because of the rigors of package handling. Items should be arranged so that all surfaces are exposed to the sterilant. Circulation of the sterilant needs to be assured on all surfaces. The trays used will have instructions, but a good rule of thumb is an inch in between each item to be sterilized in peel packs and while flashing. Sterilization indicators should be inside and outside each pack. A general rule of thumb is that the item remains sterile after proper sterilization unless the pack gets wet or is penetrated and the package is compromised. Never reuse an item meant for single use only. Monitor each load and item with mechanical indicators of time, temperature, pressure and chemical methods such as an internal or external indicator. Use biological indicators at least weekly. Very carefully clean patient care items with water and preferably an enzymatic cleaner prior to sterilization or high-level disinfection. Manually clean or use a mechanical cleaner like an ultrasonic cleaner, washer-disinfector, or washer-sterilizer as soon as you can after use. Follow the instrument instructions on the proper method of cleaning/disinfecting/sterilizing.

OSHA

OSHA (Occupational, Safety, and Health Administration) is concerned with the healthcare and other occupational hazards and procedures.

In healthcare, hazards can be found with the antiseptics, disinfectants, sterilants, and even patients. OSHA has a number of rules and regulations for healthcare. MSDS (Material Safety Data Sheets) need to be at the worksite of healthcare facilities for any chemical and substance at the site. The sheets contain information on the substance and how long the exposure time should be at the maximum.

The National Institute for Occupational Safety and Health (NIOSH) develops recommended exposure effects or systemic absorption, but not airborne substances. The American Conference on Governmental Industrial Hygienists (ACGIN) also provides guidelines on exposure limits also. It seems a bit duplicative, and in some instances, it is. Some states have their own regulations. The best thing to do is to go with the most stringent rule of all the agencies.

Detection

Organisms that are resistant to disinfection and sanitization are concerning in health care. Routine disinfection methods should be sufficient in most cases. The disinfection has to include all surfaces of the item or the organism will be hanging around for a suitable host to carry it along.

Aside from the transmission, there are methods used to find if there are organisms present on an object. Using a fluorescent marker on the object, swabbing, and culturing are used. Culturing is being used less now because of the swabbing method. The swabbing method doesn't tell what the organism is, just how many organisms are on the item, good or bad. The machine isn't that expensive for healthcare facilities when considering what data is received.

Blood Spills

Blood spills can be intimidating. Using an EPA registered tuberculocidal disinfectant should sufficiently handle the spill. Small spills on noncritical surfaces, can be disinfected with a 1:100 dilution of 5.25%-6.15% sodium hypochlorite (bleach). Large spills have to be cleaned or picked up with an absorbent prior to disinfecting, then the disinfectant or 1:10 concentration of household bleach is applied. Careful with the bleach because it is very corrosive to some materials.

Illegal drug use and needles come with their own problems. Self-disinfection of the needles can be accomplished with full strength bleach only when no needle exchange programs exist in that area. Bleach can penetrate most biofilm at full strength.

Clostridium difficile

Clostridium difficile is caused by a spore forming organism. Regular cleaning agents do not inactivate the spores of Clostridium difficile (C-diff). Most of the time health care personnel are seen as the carriers of C-Diff. The use of waterless hand sanitizers can inadvertently spread C-Diff because the organism is not truly inactivated by these products. Should an item in the room of a patient infected with C-Diff become contaminated and then touched by someone that uses waterless hand sanitizer when leaving the room, it then can be further spread to others via the hands of that healthcare person. C-Diff is a pretty hardy organism with carpets easily becoming contaminated. Even though organisms don't jump up, they can become mobile on the wheels of wheelchairs, gurneys, and even shoes. Healthcare workers often leave their shoes at the door of their home so that there is no chance of pathogen transmission to their families.

Some types of detergents actually increase the production of spores from C-Diff making its control sometimes difficult. Many large facilities are becoming more aware of the transmission of C-Diff and because of this, they are disinfecting rooms of patients with C-Diff with a chlorine solution. The chlorine solution has proven to be more effective than using quaternary ammonium products.

The effective eradication of C-Diff transmission within healthcare facilities often requires a multi-modal approach. Hand washing versus waterless hand sanitizer along with barrier precautions and a disinfection with chlorine have proven to be effective.

Cryptosporidium is resistant to chlorine at normal concentrations not used for disinfection. C. parvum is not completely inactivated by most disinfectants used in healthcare including ethyl alcohol, and quaternary ammonium compounds. The only chemical disinfectants and sterilants able to inactivate a lot of C. parvum were 6% and 7.5% hydrogen peroxide. Sterilization methods will fully inactivate C. parvum, including steam, EtO, and hydrogen peroxide gas plasma. Although most disinfectants are ineffective against C. parvum, current cleaning and disinfection practices appear satisfactory to prevent healthcare-associated transmission.

Inactivation of Bioterrorist Agents

Publications have highlighted concerns about the potential for biological terrorism. The CDC has categorized several agents as "high priority" because they can be easily disseminated or transmitted from person to person, cause high mortality, and are likely to cause public panic and social disruption.

These agents include Bacillus anthracis (the cause of anthrax), Yersinia pestis (plague), variola major (smallpox), Clostridium botulinum toxin (botulism), Francisella tularensis (tularemia), filoviruses (Ebola hemorrhagic fever, Marburg hemorrhagic fever); and arenaviruses (Lassa [Lassa fever], Junin [Argentine hemorrhagic fever]), and related viruses.

Many of the bioterrorism agents can be disinfected and sterilized in the normal manner. They are also transmitted the same way that other organisms are transmitted, including airborne. Spores would be the most difficult to disinfect or sterilize.

Conclusion

The proper use of disinfection and sterilization will save funds from lawsuits and follow up of contaminated item events. Always remember to clean prior to disinfection and clean meticulously. This is a short guide to make disinfection and sterilization easy for the reader to understand. There are many more thorough books, however, getting the information out and in easy to understand terms was most important. Following are some pictures of both good and bad outcomes of sterilization and ways of cleaning and keeping offices. Sterilization was left to the end of the document due to its importance. Always check with your State Quality Improvement Unit or Surveyors for particular questions or advice. They are there to help along with survey.

Picture Examples

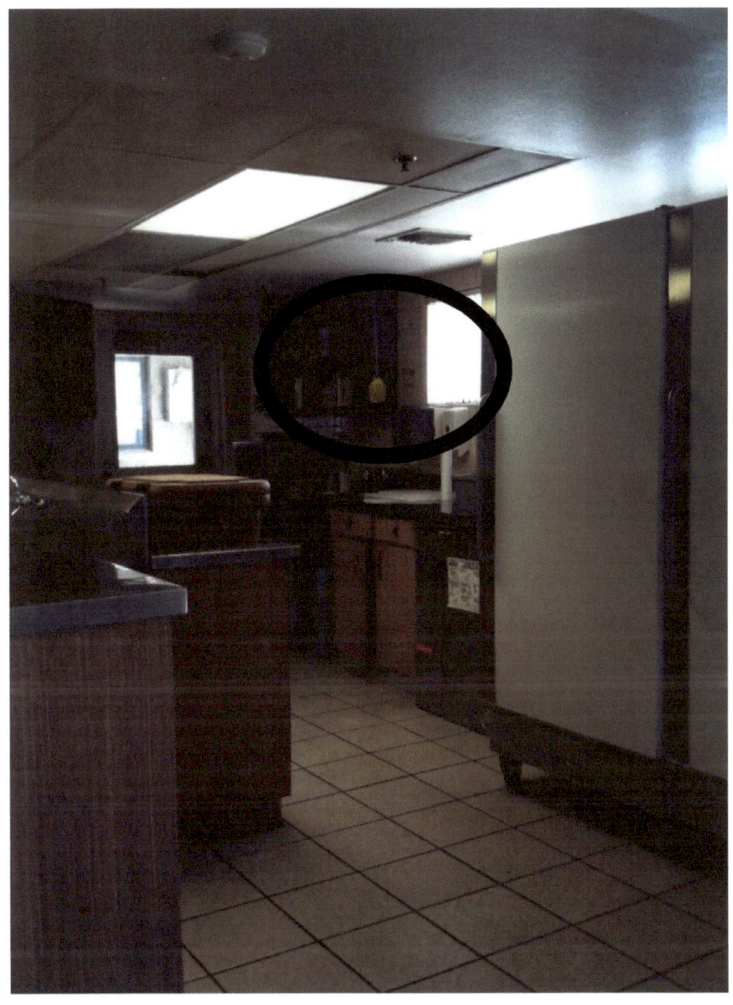

Healthcare facilities don't put flyswatters out (look above the sink)

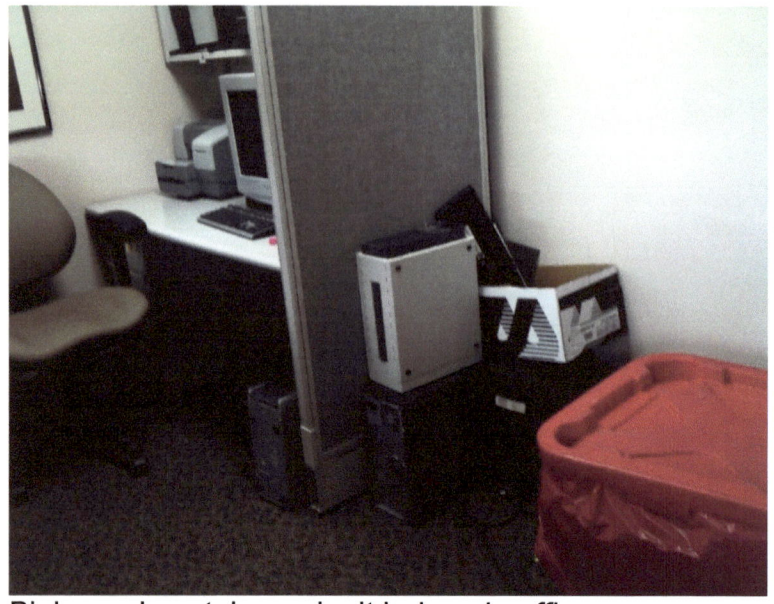

Biohazard containers don't belong in offices

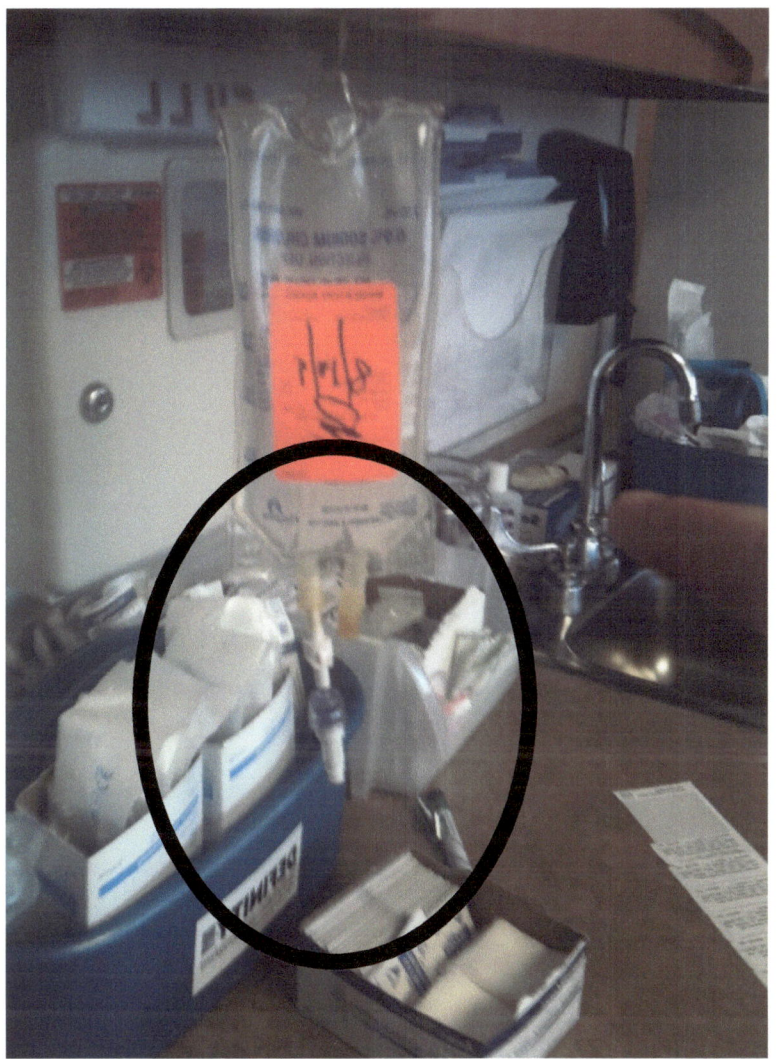

IV solutions should never be used over and over as saline flushes

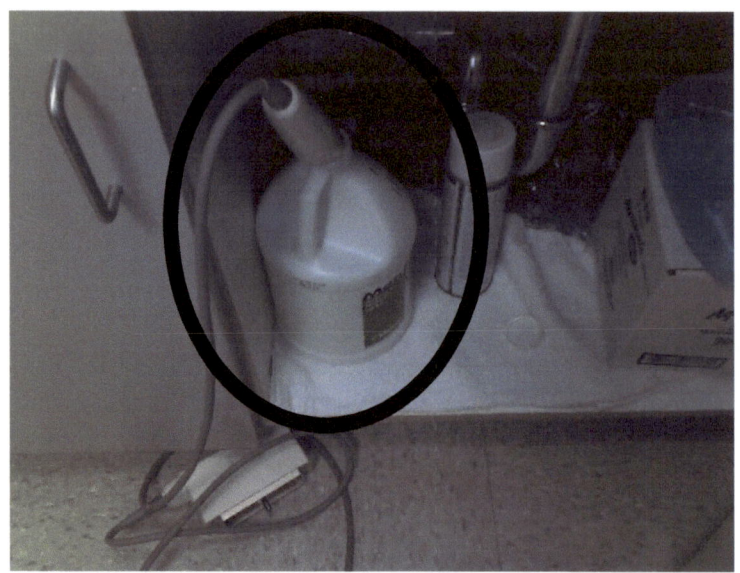

Ultrasonic probes should never be stuck in a disinfectant like this, it should be cleaned, disinfected and hung dry. Plus, it shouldn't be under a sink.

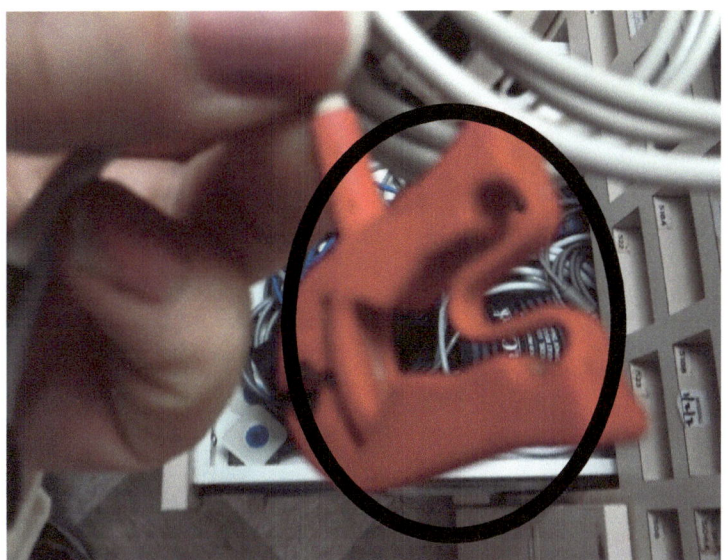

EKG snaps should be cleaned and wiped down between patients, don't let scum accumulate

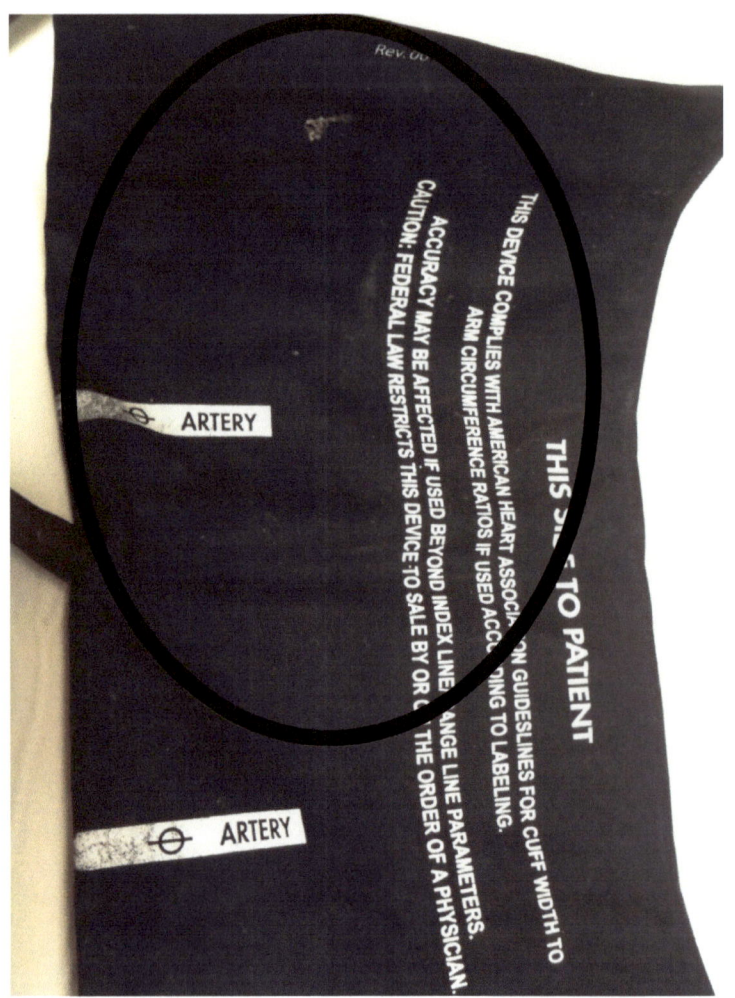

Scum should not be on reusable BP cuffs, they should be cleaned at least daily

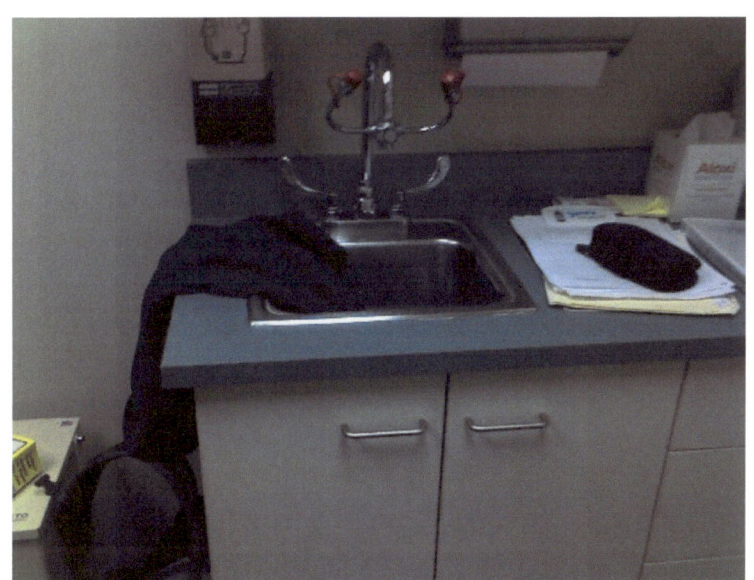

A sweater should not be on a procedure sink, it should be in the employee lounge or office.

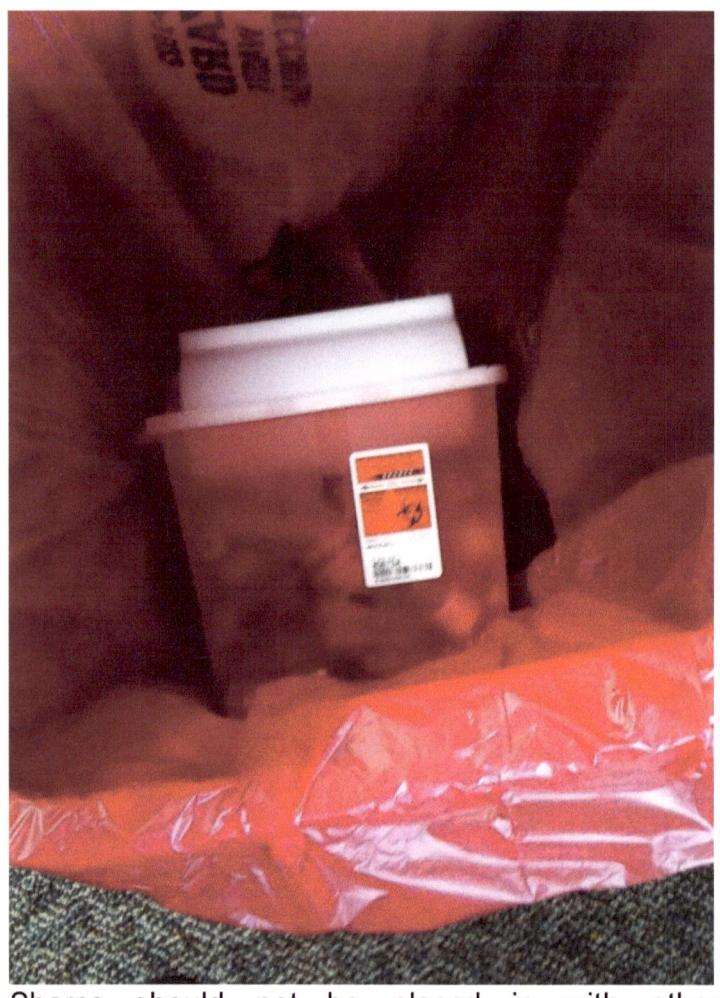

Sharps should not be placed in with other biohazardous waste

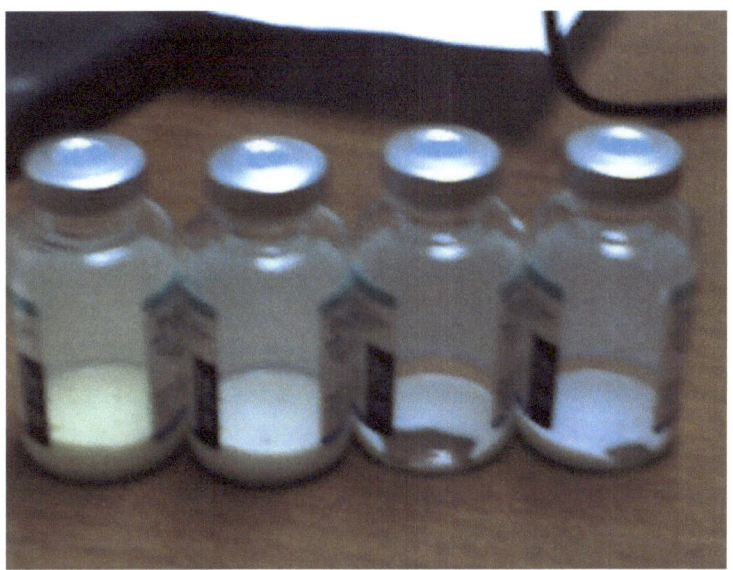

Once used, toss profofol containers, they degrade when oxygen is present and should not be reused anyway. The medication should be wasted prior to placing in a biohazardous sharps container.

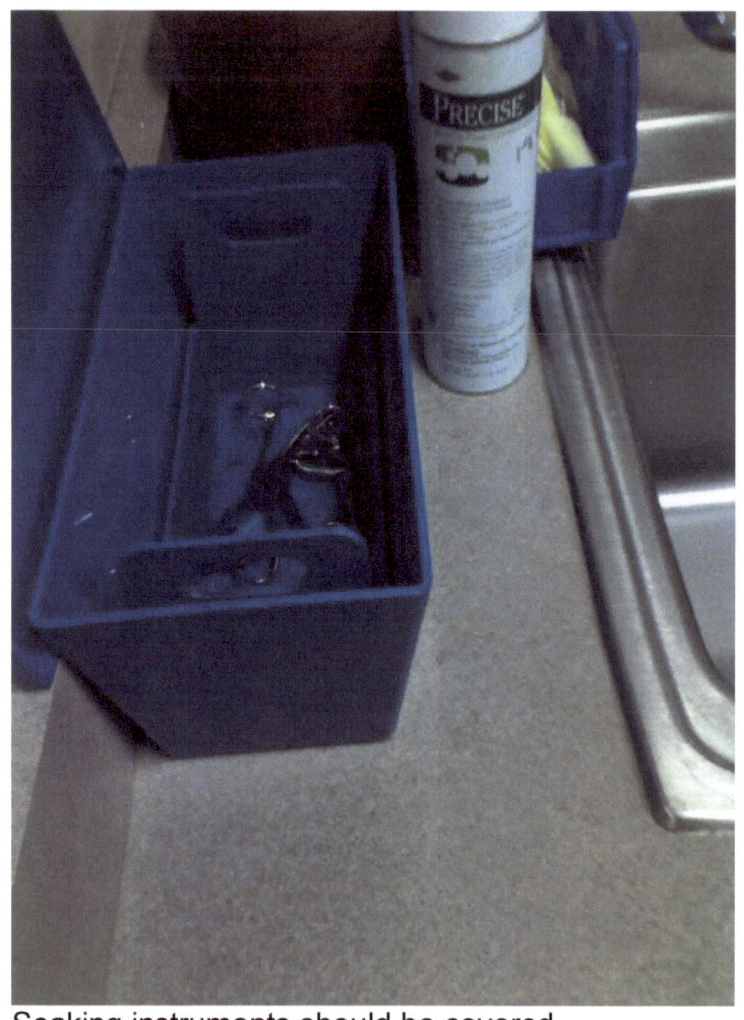

Soaking instruments should be covered

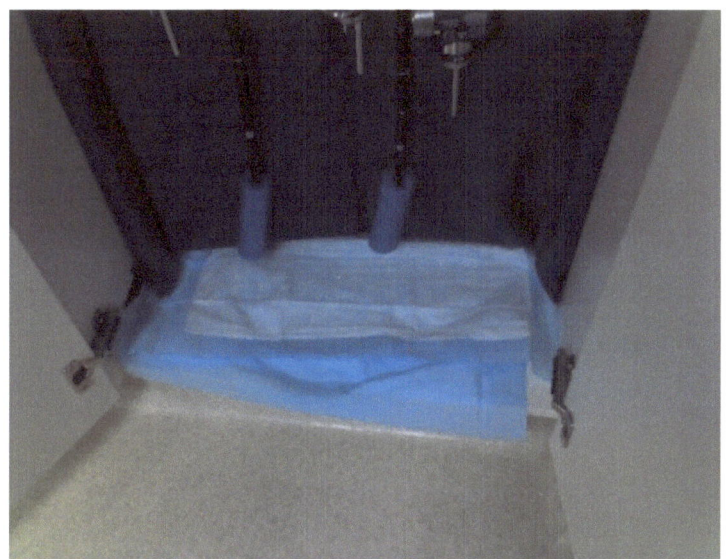

Pad under hanging endoscopes indicates wet scopes were put away

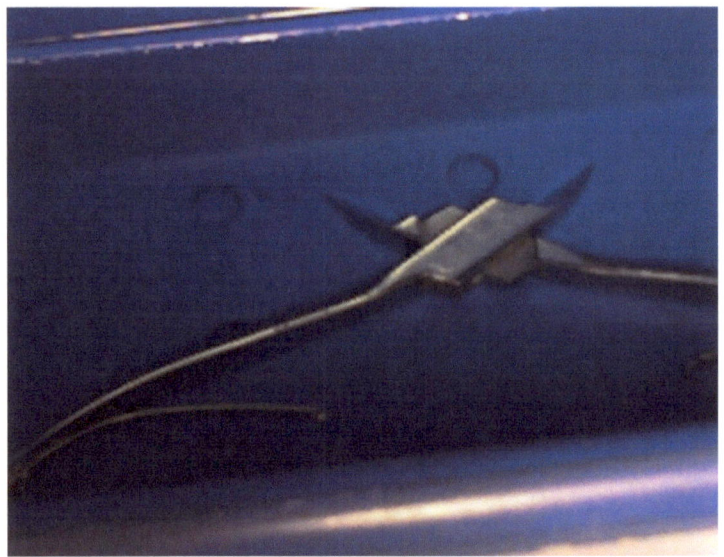

Correct soaking of instrument, needs covered also with lid

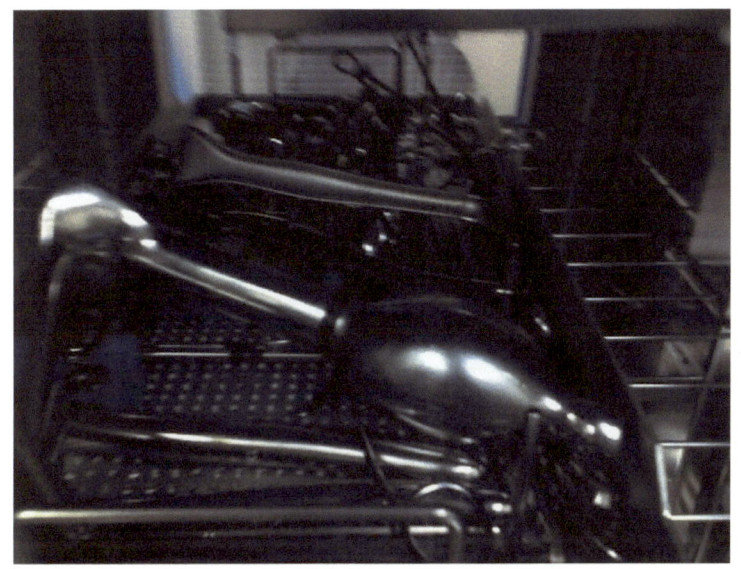

Overloaded washer with instruments not open

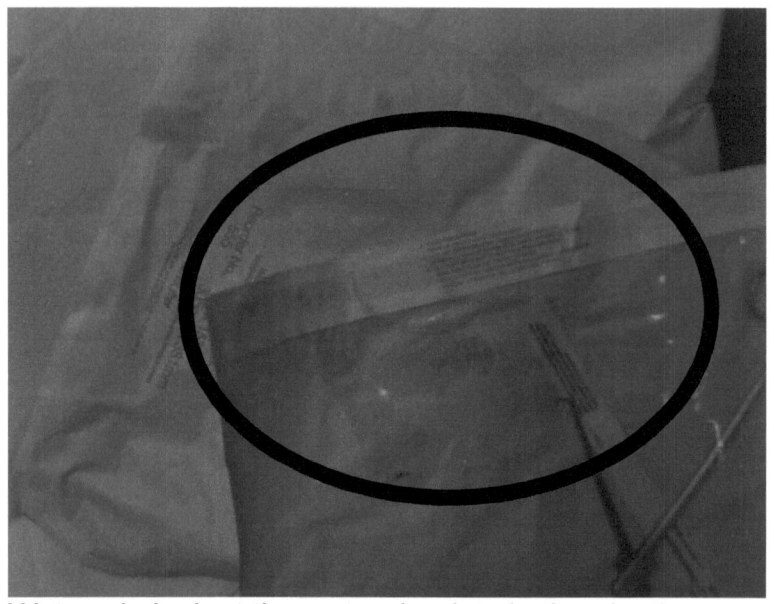

Wet pack, look at the water droplets in the plastic

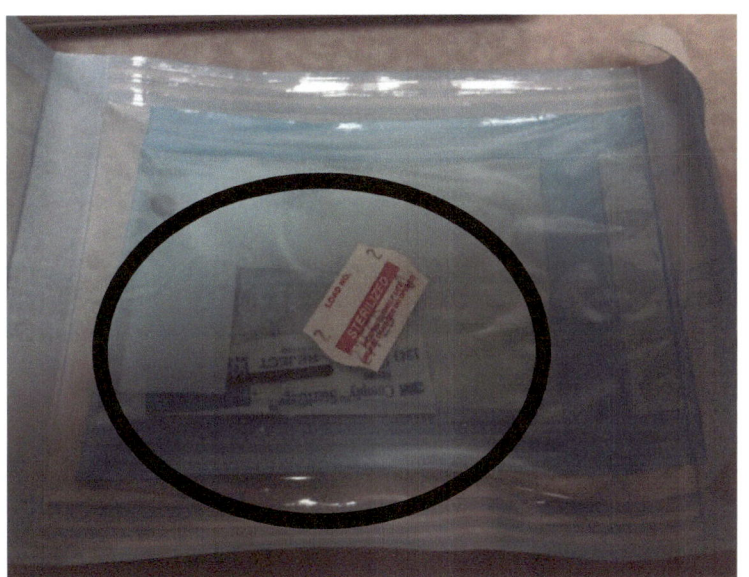

Internal and external indicator present, notice the reject indicator

69

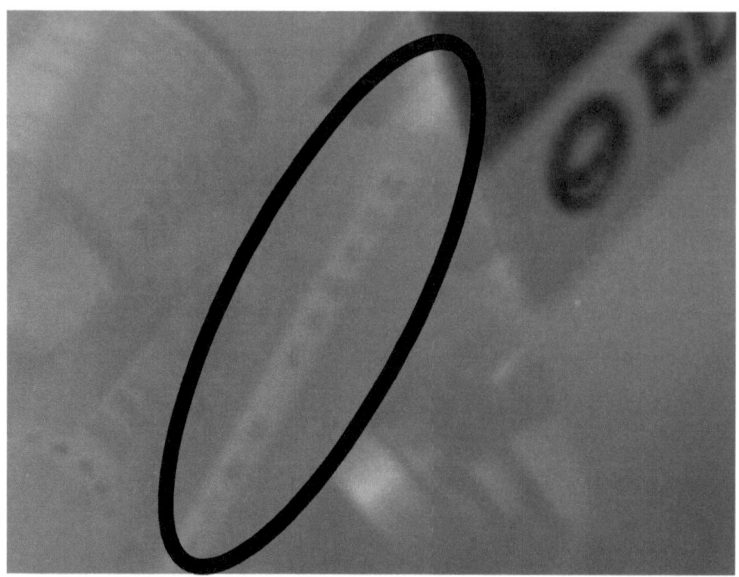

Syringes and ampules and vials should be empty prior to placing in sharps container

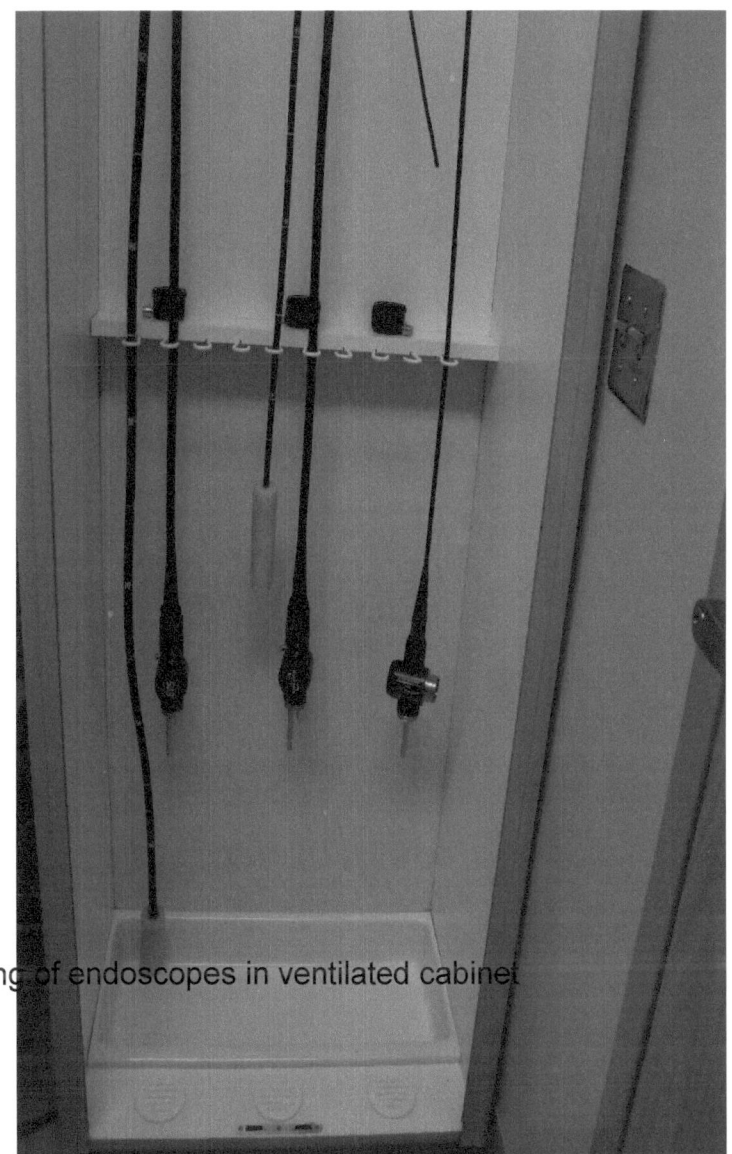

Proper hanging of endoscopes in ventilated cabinet

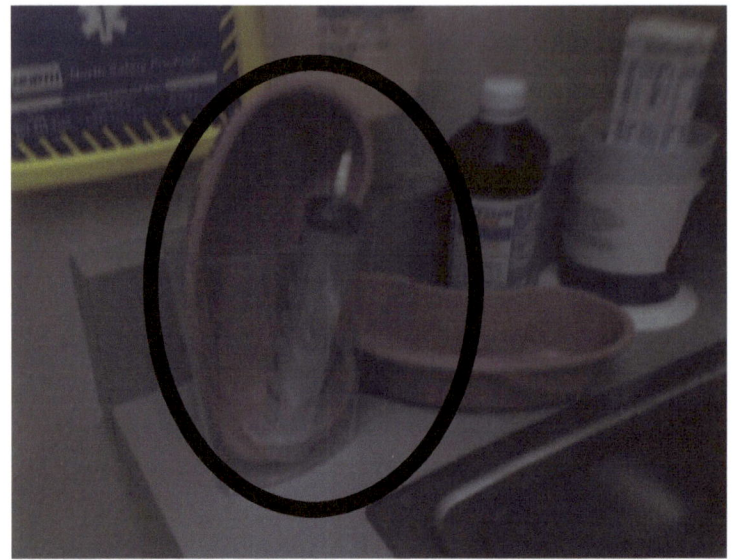

Ear flushers are not to be used more than once, single use only

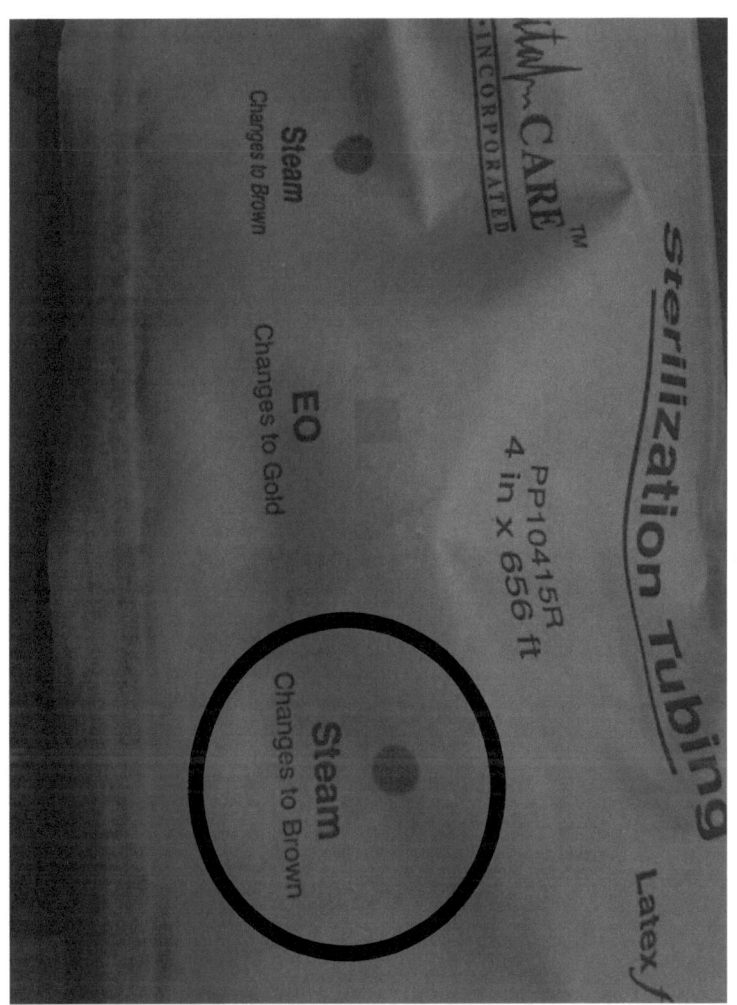

This was put out to use on a patient, pink dot under steam indicated not-sterile

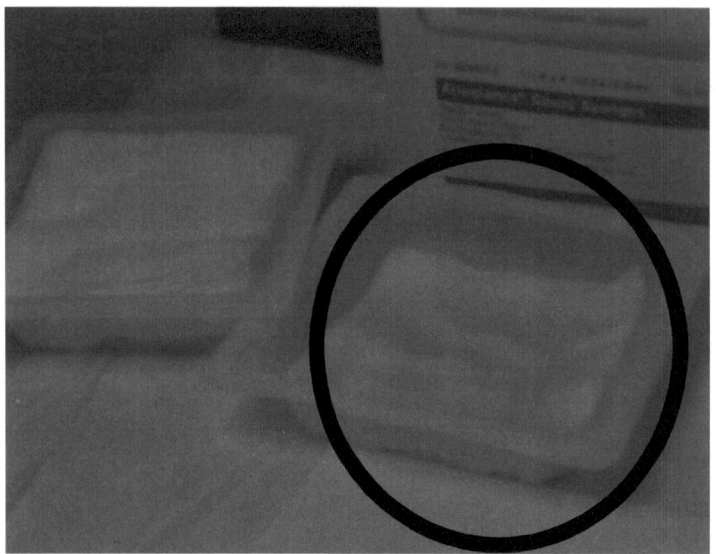

Pre-moistened gauze should not be used on multiple patients

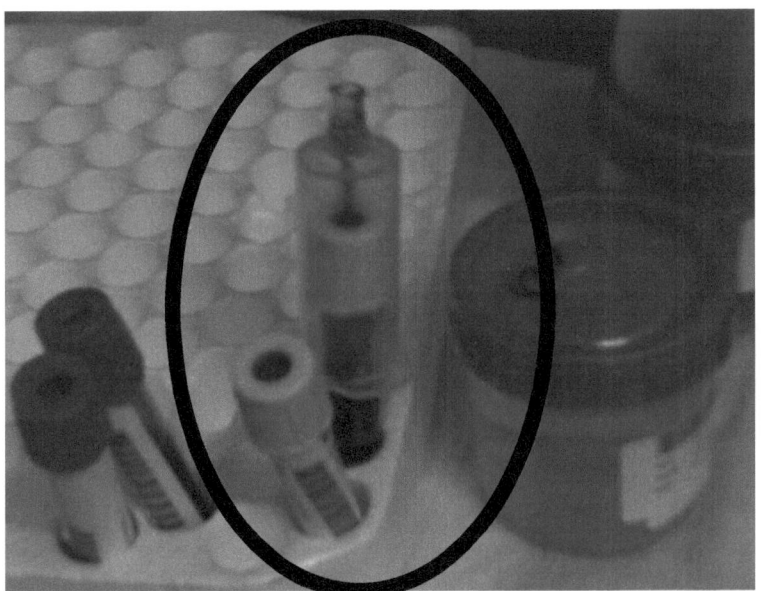
Vacutainers should not be stored with injector on, one bump and an exposure to blood can occur

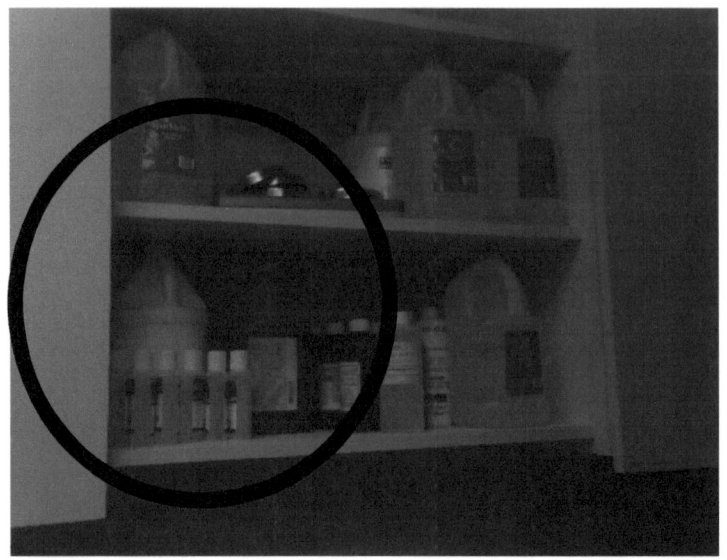

Medications should not be stored with disinfectants or potable water

Syringes with unlabeled medication should not be stored, notice no med name

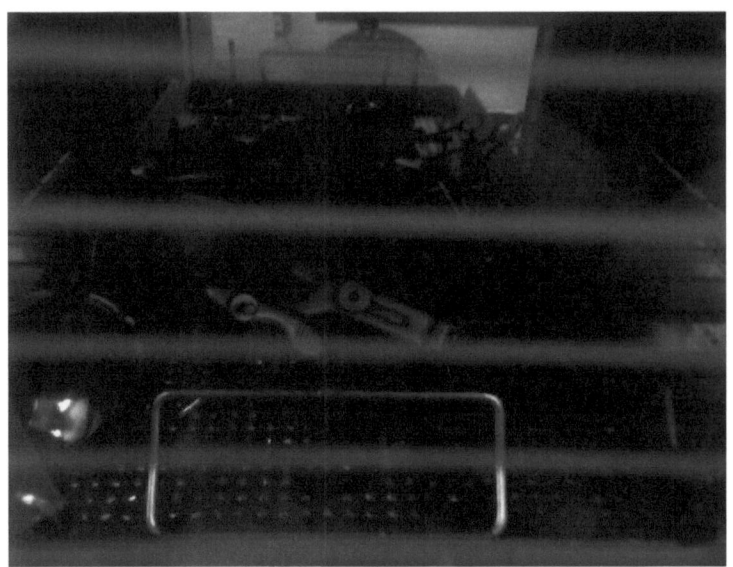

Very overloaded washer/disinfector

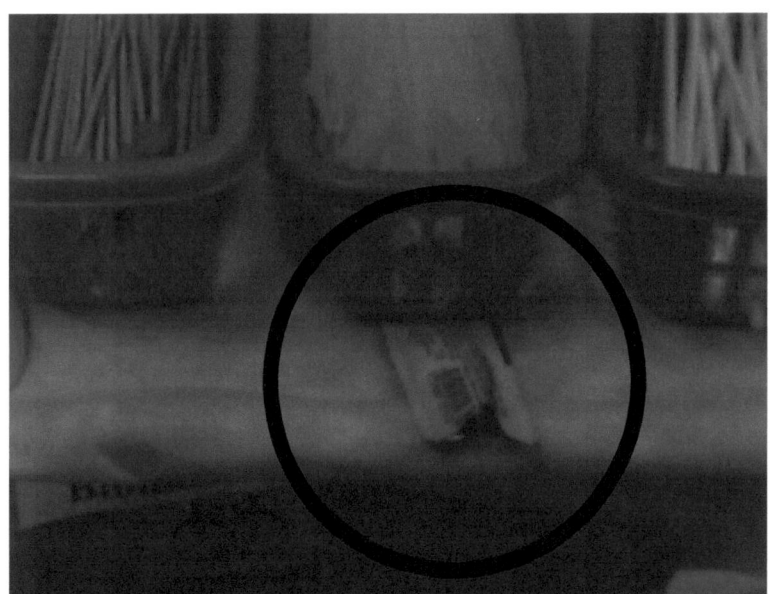

Lubricant tube is not to be reused patient to patient,
this one is single use only

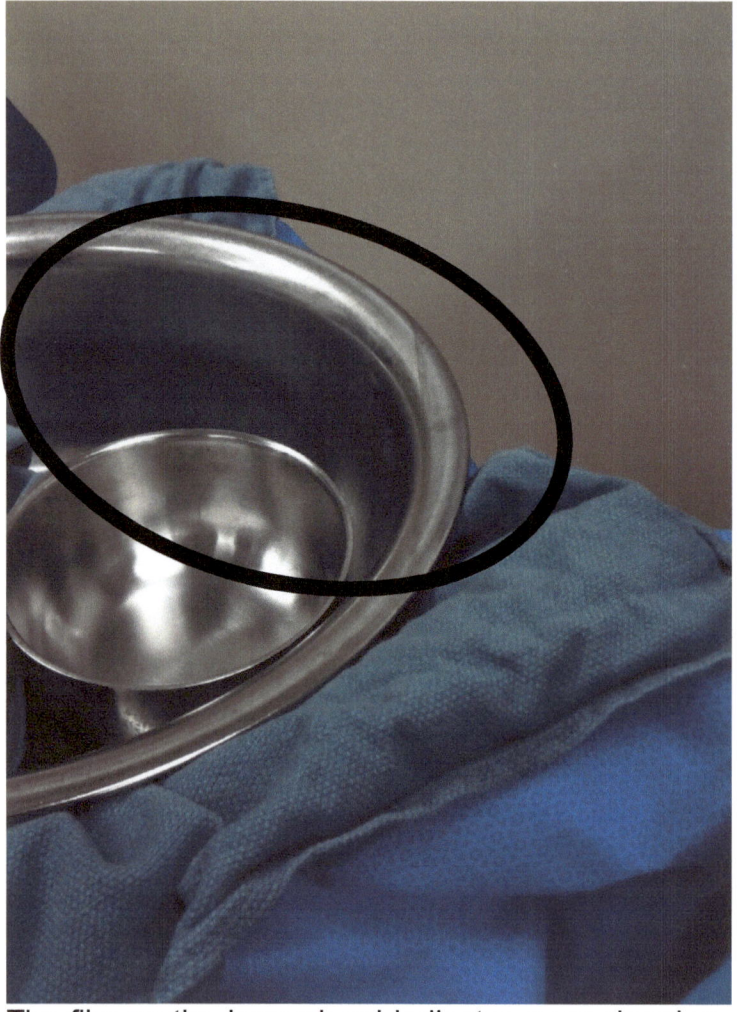

The film on the larger bowl indicates poor cleaning prior to sterilization

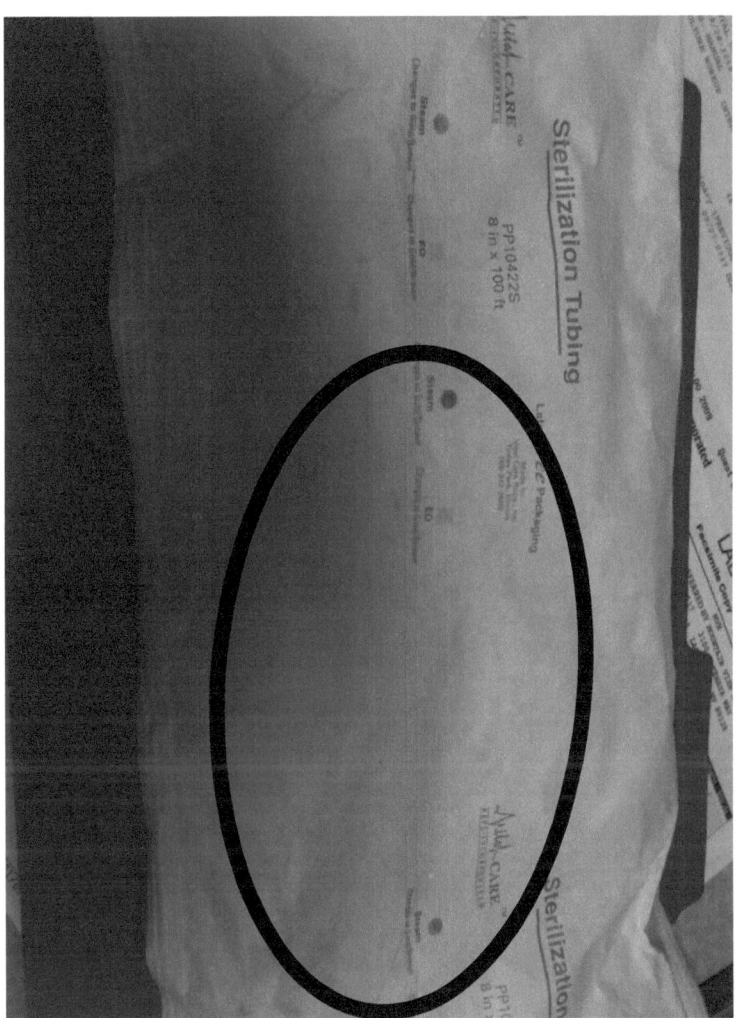

Wet pack, see the water stains on the white outer wrap

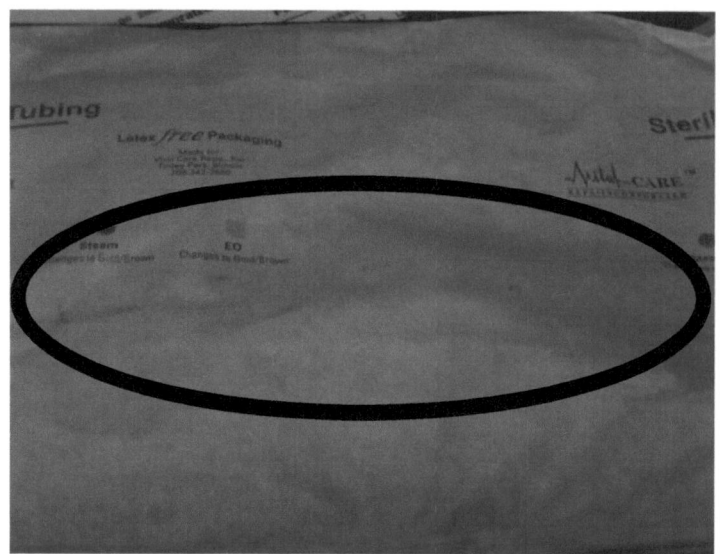

Indicator says sterile, however pack has water stains on it making it a wet pack

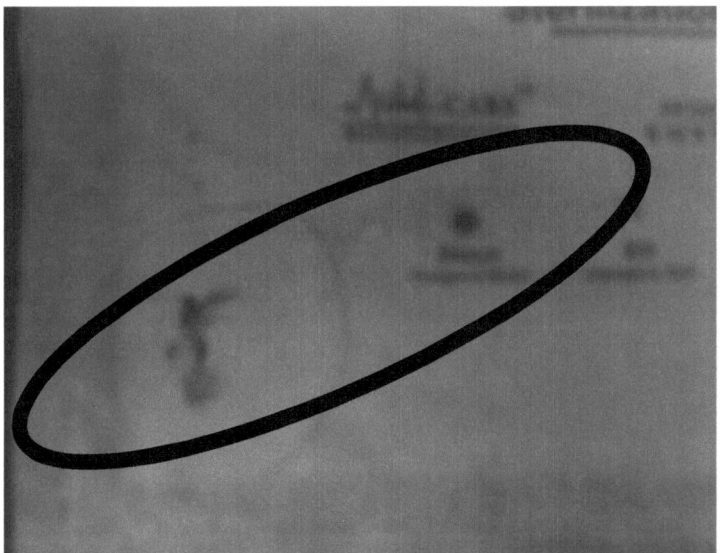

Wet pack indicated by blue stain on wrapper from overloaded steam sterilizer. Notice the positive indicator on the wrap indicating the sterilizer got up to the proper temperature.

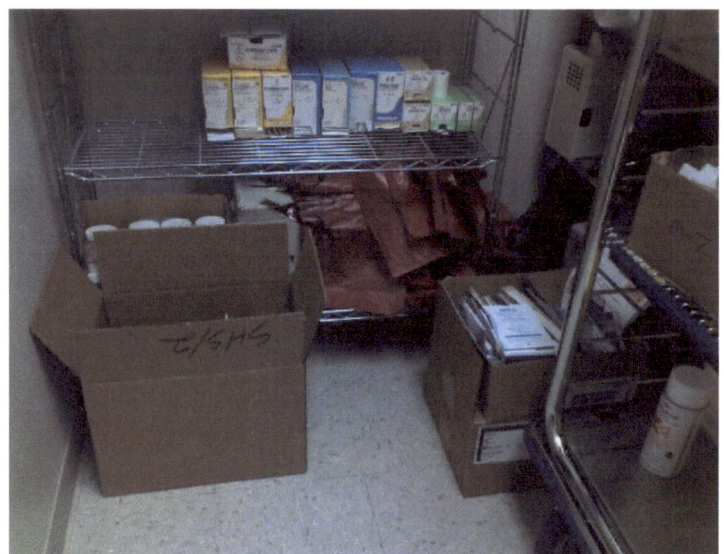

Storage cabinets should be well organized, not like this. Suture material should not be stored with disinfectants like the one in the can on the right.

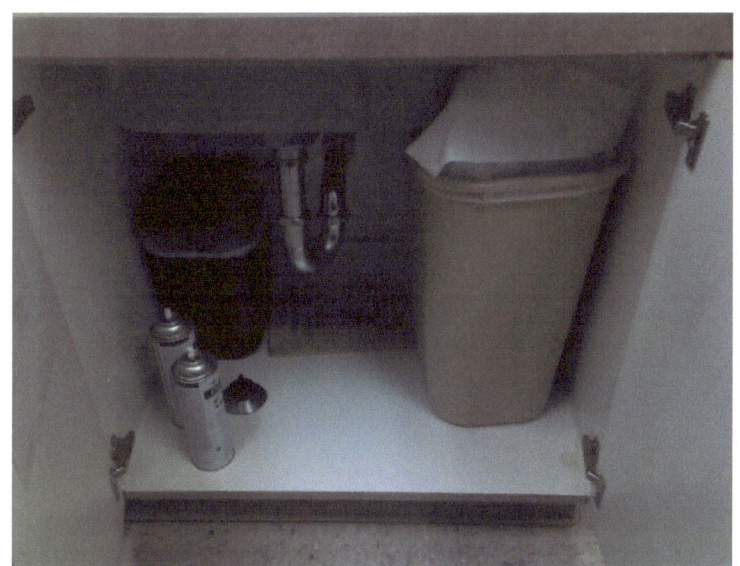

Nothing should be stored under sinks

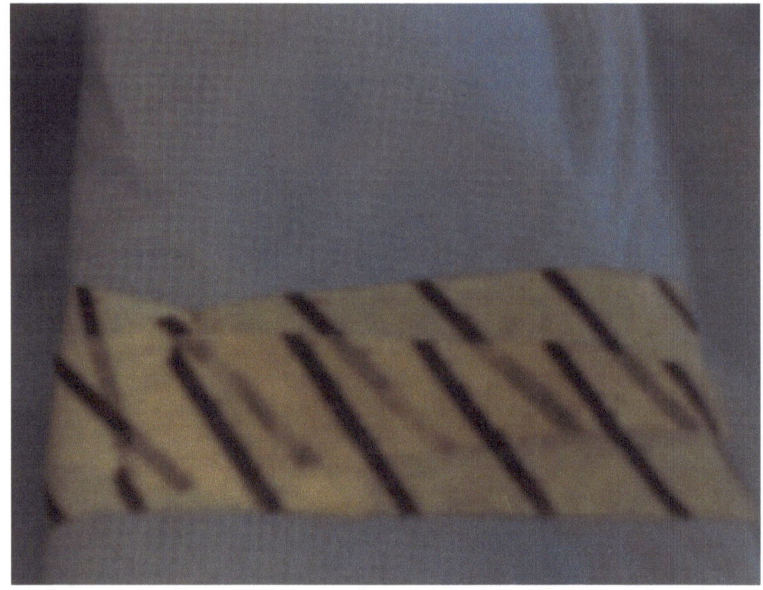

External indicator tape should have dark strips to
indicate temperature was reached for sterilization

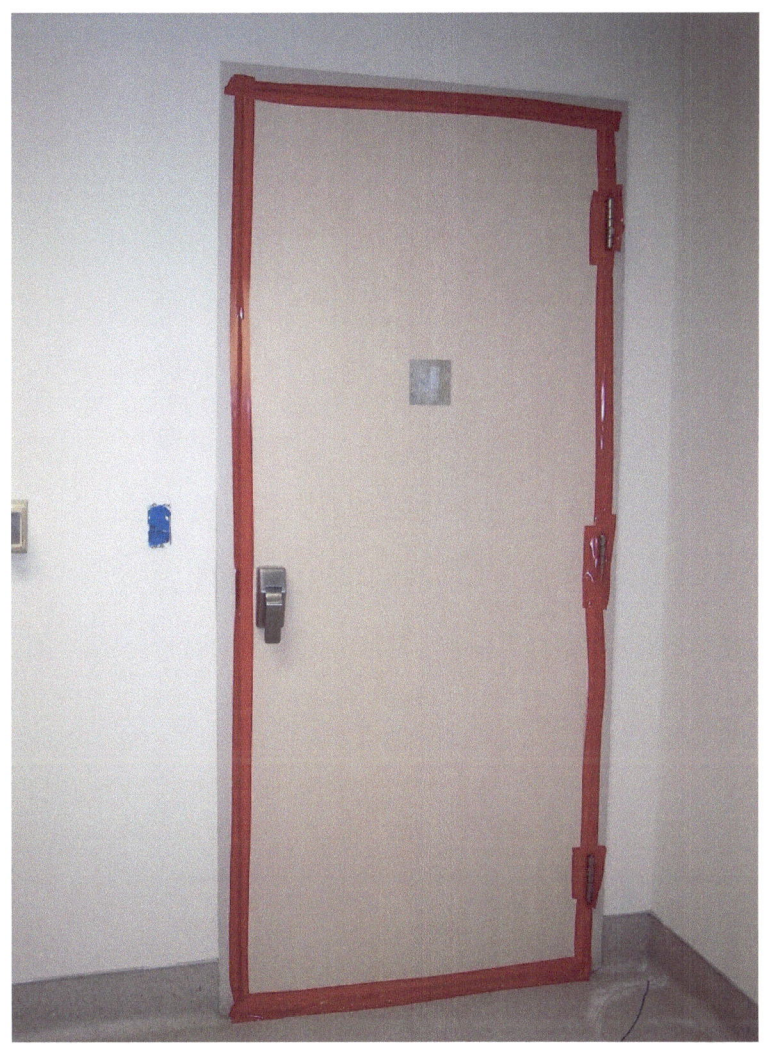

Construction should be completely isolated from other areas

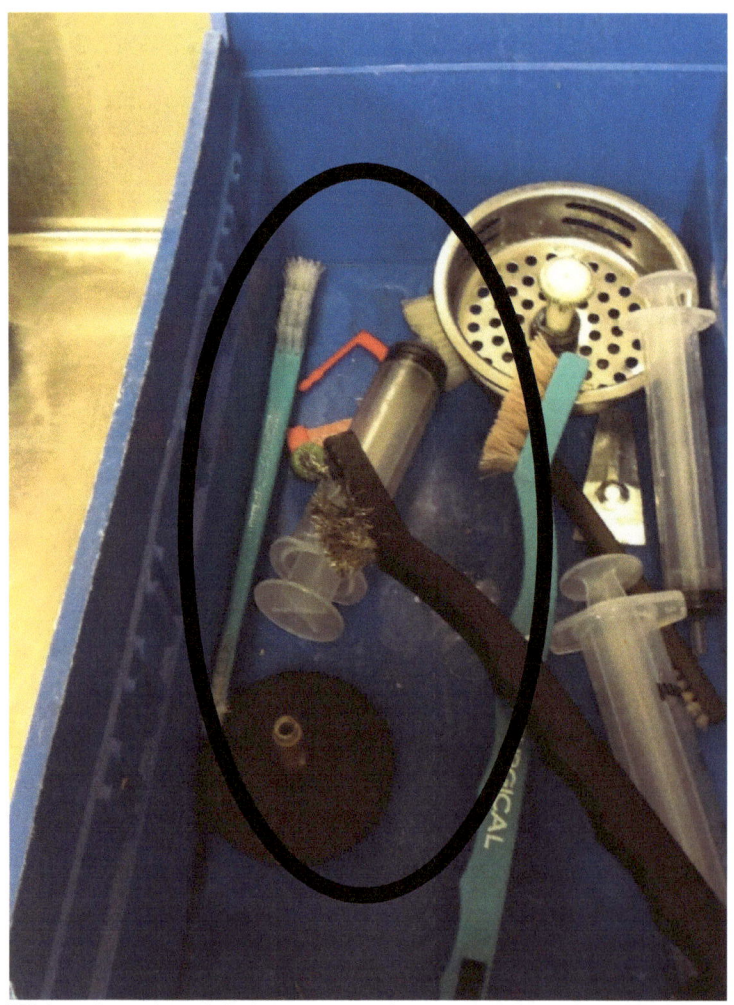

This cleaning kit is gross, the steel brush probably can't clean anything and the other brushes are tattered

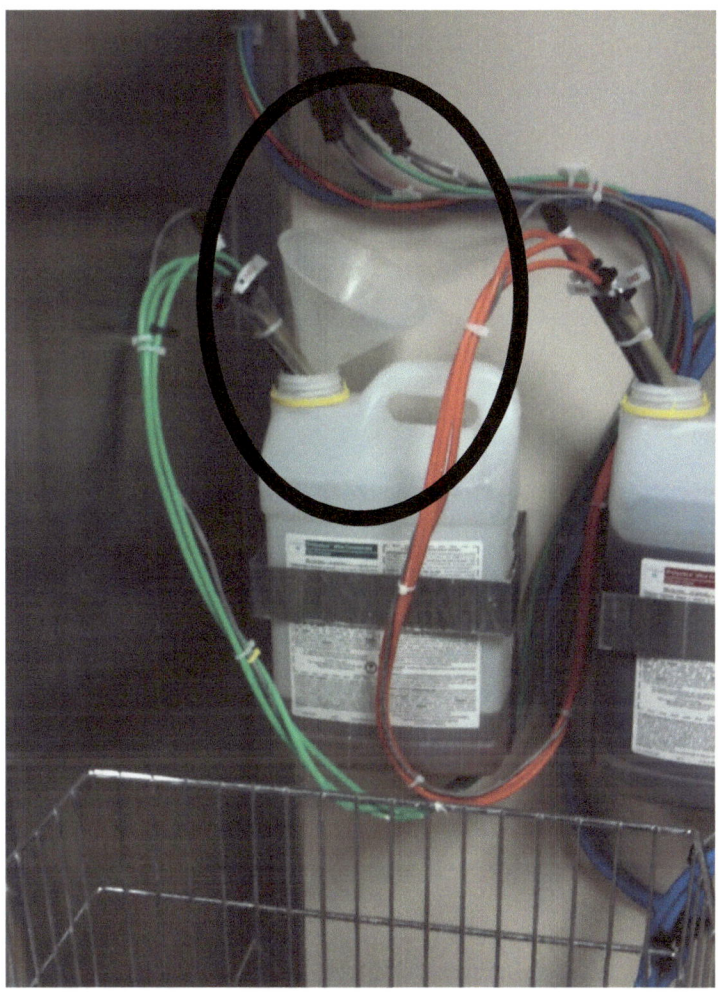

Refilling disinfector containers is not good practice (notice the funnel)

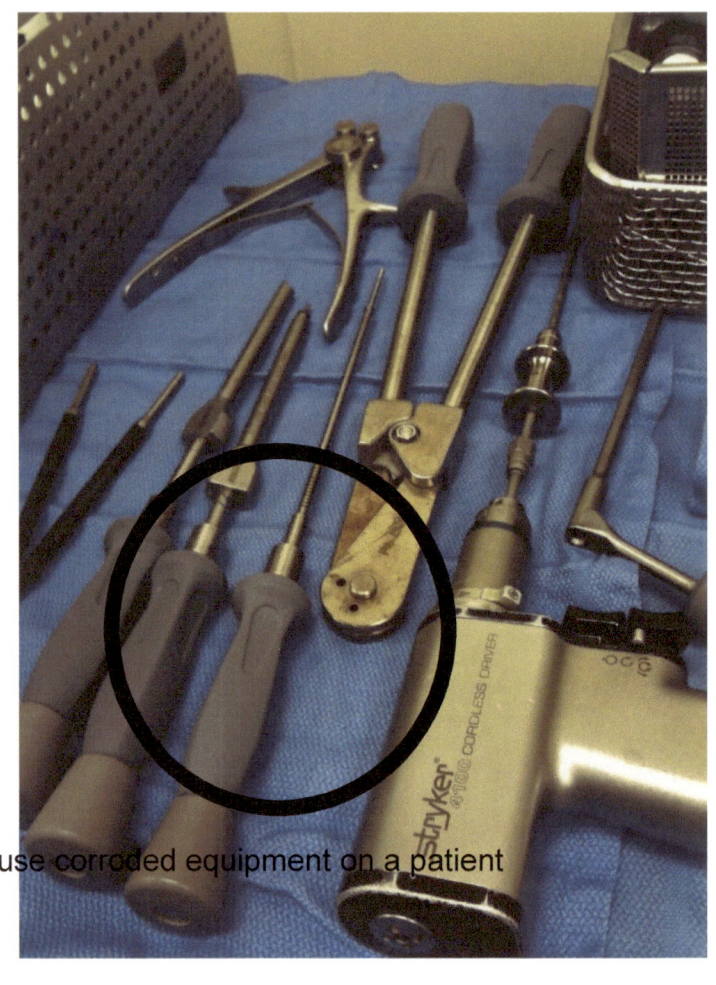
Never use corroded equipment on a patient

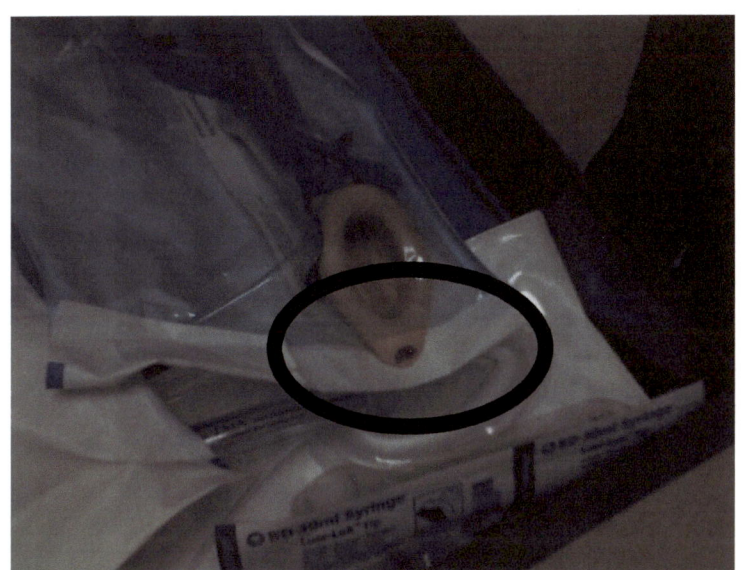

Airway supposed to be sterile, but protruding through sterile pack so not sterile

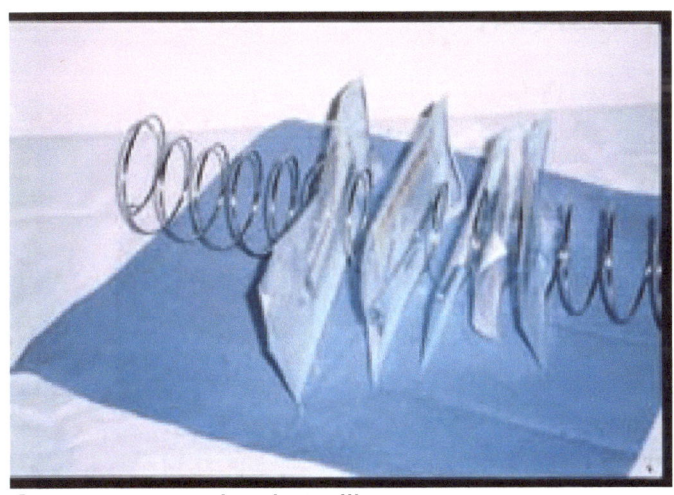

Correct way to load sterilizer

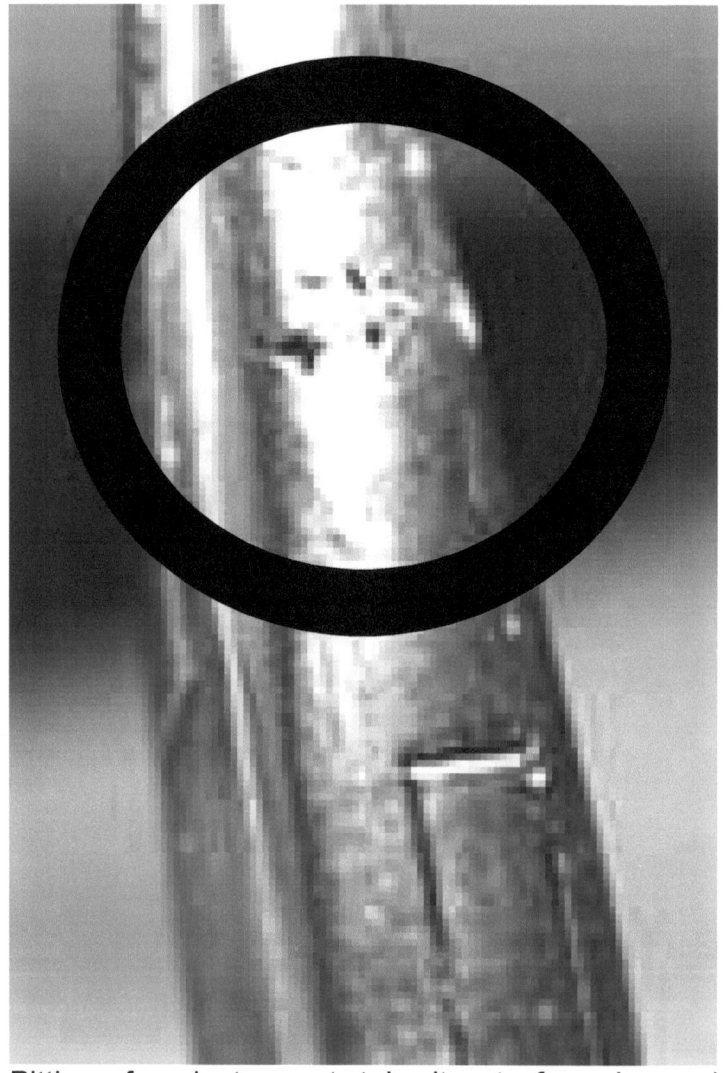

Pitting of an instrument, take it out of service and replace

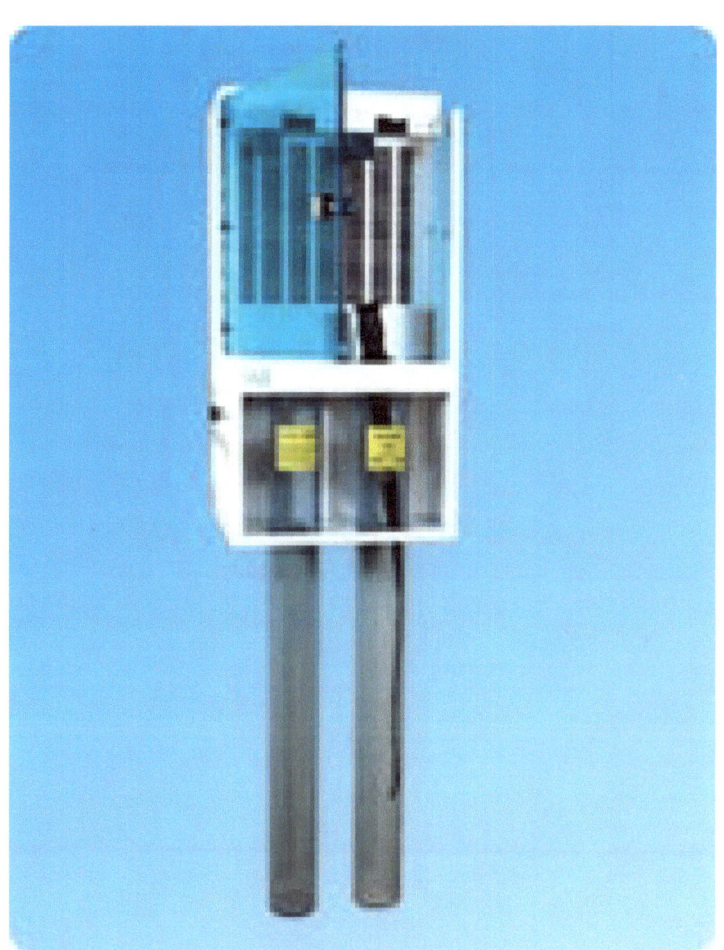

Correct storage for urological scopes

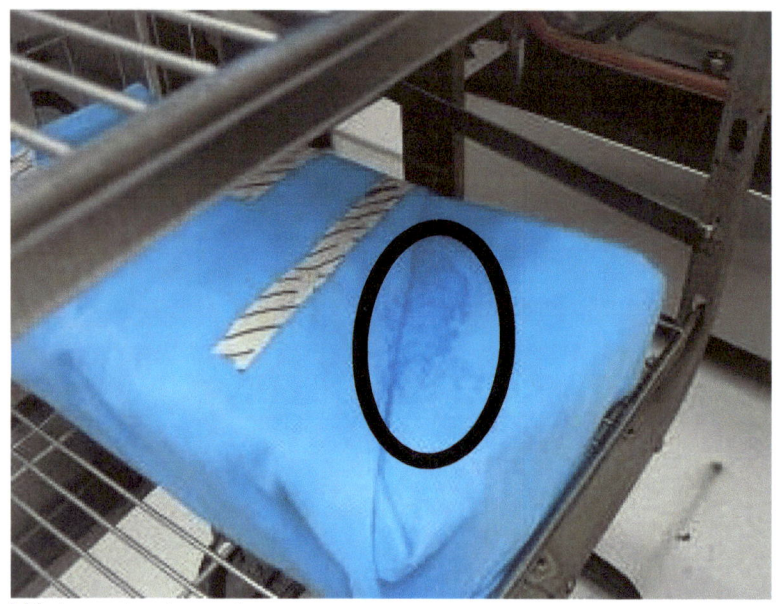

Wet pack, do not use

www.ingramcontent.com/pod-product-compliance
Lightning Source LLC
Chambersburg PA
CBHW040827180526
45159CB00001B/98